ACTA NEUROCHIRURGICA / SUPPLEMENTUM X

DIE KLASSIFIKATION DER HIRNTUMOREN

BERICHT ÜBER DAS INTERNATIONALE SYMPOSION
IN KÖLN VOM 30. AUGUST BIS 1. SEPTEMBER 1961

UNTER FÖRDERUNG DURCH
DIE MAX-PLANCK-GESELLSCHAFT
DIE DEUTSCHE FORSCHUNGSGEMEINSCHAFT UND
DIE WORLD FEDERATION OF NEUROLOGY

HERAUSGEGEBEN VON

K. J. ZÜLCH UND A. L. WOOLF
KÖLN · SMETHWICK

MIT 71 TEXTABBILDUNGEN

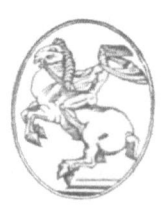

WIEN / SPRINGER-VERLAG / 1964

ACTA NEUROCHIRURGICA / SUPPLEMENTUM X

CLASSIFICATION
OF BRAIN TUMOURS

REPORT OF THE INTERNATIONAL SYMPOSIUM
AT COLOGNE 30th AUGUST — 1st SEPTEMBER 1961

SPONSORED BY

THE MAX-PLANCK-GESELLSCHAFT
THE DEUTSCHE FORSCHUNGSGEMEINSCHAFT AND
THE WORLD FEDERATION OF NEUROLOGY

EDITED BY

K. J. ZÜLCH AND A. L. WOOLF
COLOGNE   SMETHWICK

WITH 71 FIGURES

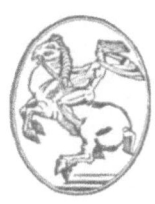

VIENNA / SPRINGER-VERLAG / 1964

ISBN 978-3-211-80712-5   ISBN 978-3-7091-5820-3 (eBook)
DOI 10.1007/978-3-7091-5820-3

Preface

The report which follows constitutes the proceedings of a symposium on the classification of brain tumours held in Cologne in 1961. It contains the contributions and discussions reported as far· as possible in a word-for-word manner, in the hope not only of providing out of the thoughts of the participants stimulation for further research, but also to indicate the atmosphere which prevailed during the symposium in which many completely opposed views were able to be expressed without any feeling of embarrassment. This freedom of expression is already obvious in the discussion of a proposed classification of brain tumours for the Unio Internationalis Contra Cancrum (UICC). The symposium endeavoured here to produce a positive criticism in order to arrive at a significant and practical conclusion viz a general, internationally acceptable classification. It was necessary to accept a degree of compromise even if the classification suggested did not in every point correspond to all the personal views of the various participants.

The second part of the symposium was concerned with a critical discussion of numerous brain tumour problems, for example the scientific delineation of tumour groups; the discussion was started by general reviews on the biology of brain tumours so that the later discussion could cover as wide a ground as possibly. Here also we all felt that a great stimulus for future work arose from the discussion.

The contributions of the individual participants could be presented in the original form with illustrations. In the discussion it has only been necessary to discard obvious repetitions or errors of speech otherwise as far as possible a word-for-word rendering has been made with the help of tape recording. As all the participants were fluent in English, the proceedings have been recorded in this language so that as wide a possible distribution of the contents may be obtained.

We have to thank the editor and publishers of Acta Neurochirurgica for making possible the publication to a wide audience. We are also indebted to Dr. *Lüthy* and Frau *Kortekamp* for their skilled deciphering of the discussion recorded on tape.

The participants in the symposium have later come together as the Working Group for Neuro-oncology in the World Federation of Neurology. We hope that this first fruitful symposium will be followed regularly by others and in conclusion thank once more the organisations who have made possible the symposium: the Deutsche Forschungsgemeinschaft, the World Federation of Neurology and the Max-Planck Society.

November 1963.

K. J. Zülch, Cologne   *A. L. Woolf, Smethwick*

Vorwort

Der vorliegende Bericht gibt die Verhandlungen eines Symposions in Köln 1961 über die Klassifikation der Hirngeschwülste wieder. Er enthält die Vorträge und Diskussionen in möglichst wortgetreuer Form in der Hoffnung, aus den Gedanken der Teilnehmer Anregungen für die weitere Forschung zu geben, aber auch um den Geist der Zusammenarbeit zu zeigen, der die Teilnehmer selbst bei völlig gegensätzlicher Meinung in dieser Aussprache leitete. Diese Einstellung zeigte sich bereits bei der Besprechung eines Klassifikationsvorschlages der Hirntumoren der Unio Internationalis Contra Cancrum (UICC). Das Symposion versuchte hier eine positive Kritik, um dies bedeutsame und praktisch erreichbare Ziel zu fördern: eine allgemeine, international annehmbare Klassifikation zu schaffen. Ein solcher Kompromiß schien wichtig, selbst wenn das vorgesehene Schema nicht in allen Punkten der eigenen Meinung entsprechen konnte.

Der zweite Teil des Symposions diente einer kritischen Aussprache zahlreicher Fragen der Hirntumoren, unter anderem der wissenschaftlichen Abgrenzung der Geschwulstgruppen; er wurde aber durch einige allgemeine Referate über die Biologie der Hirntumoren eingeleitet, um diese Diskussion in einen möglichst breiten Rahmen zu stellen. Auch hier scheint uns aus der Diskussion eine Fülle von Anregungen für zukünftige Arbeiten hervorzugehen.

Die Referate der einzelnen Teilnehmer konnten in der breiten Originalfassung und mit Bildern wiedergegeben werden. Aus der Diskussion wurden nur offensichtliche Wiederholungen oder Sprechfehler ausgemerzt, sonst aber eine möglichst wortgetreue Wiedergabe auf Grund der Bandaufnahmen angestrebt. Da alle Teilnehmer das Englische beherrschten, wurden die Verhandlungen in dieser Sprache geführt und auch in der schriftlichen Wiedergabe beibehalten, um eine möglichst weite Verbreiterung des Inhaltes zu ermöglichen.

Wir haben Herausgeber und Verlag der Acta Neurochirurgica zu danken, die den Druck in dem breiten Rahmen möglich machten, Dr. *Lüthy* und Frau *Kortekamp* gebührt Dank für die nicht immer ganz leichte Entzifferung des Textes aus dem besprochenen Band.

Die Teilnehmer des Symposions haben sich später zur Arbeits-gemeinschaft für Neuro-Onkologie in der Weltvereinigung für Neu-rologie zusammengefunden. Wir hoffen, daß diesem ersten frucht-baren Symposion regelmäßig weitere folgen werden und danken zum Schluß noch einmal den Organisationen, die das Symposion gefördert haben: der Deutschen Forschungsgemeinschaft, der World Federation of Neurology und der Max-Planck-Gesellschaft.

November 1963.

K. J. Zülch, Köln   *A. L. Woolf,* Smethwick

Contents

Page

Zülch, K. J. Introduction 1
Zülch, K. J. The Classification of Brain Tumours 3

I. Classification of Brain Tumours
a) General Remarks on Classification
Hamperl, H. The Nomenclature of Tumours of the Nervous System 5
  Discussion 9

b) The Contribution of Different Techniques to Classification

1. *Genetics* 24
   Koch, G. The Genetics of Cerebral Tumours 24
   Discussion 28
2. *Cerebral Tumours in Animals* 30
   Luginbühl, H. A Comparative Study of Neoplasms of the Central Nervous System in Animal 30
   Discussion 42
3. *Experimental Production of Brain Tumours* 46
   Netsky, M. G. Experimental Induction and Transplantation of Brain Tumours in Animals 46
   Discussion 56
   Schiefer, B. Morphology of Experimental Brain Tumours 57
   Discussion 63
4. *Tissue Culture* 68
   Kersting, G. Tissue Culture and the Classification of Brain Tumours . . 68
   Discussion 72
5. *Electron Microscopy* 75
   Woolf, A. L. Remarks on the Electronmicroscopical Appearances of Brain Tumours 75
   Discussion 78
6. *Histochemistry* 80
   Müller, W. Remarks on the Histochemistry of Brain Tumours 80
   Discussion 84
7. *Metallic Impregnation* 85
   Calvo, W. Observations on the Metallic Impregnations of Brain Tumours 85
   Discussion 93

II. The Malignancy and Grading of Tumours
Sayre, G. P. The System of Grading of Gliomas 98
  Discussion 106
Zülch, K. J. Grading of Malignancy of Brain Tumours 117
  Discussion 119

Page

III. Spongioblastoma

Zülch, K. J. Some Remarks on the Spongioblastoma of the Brain 121
    Discussion 125
Rubinstein, L. J. Discussion on Polar Spongioblastomas 126
    Discussion 132

IV. Polymorphous Oligodendroglioma

Rubinstein, L. J. Morphological Problems of Brain Tumours with Mixed
    Cell Population 141
    Discussion 158
Zülch, K. J. On the Definition of the Polymorphous Oligodendroglioma . . 166
    Discussion 168
Luginbühl, H. Oligodendrogliomas in Animals 173
    Discussion 181

V. Sarcoma and Related Processes

Zülch, K. J. Primary Sarcomas of the Brain 185
Bingas, B. On the Primary Sarcomas of the Brain 186
Brucher, J. M. The Classification and Diagnosis of Intracranial Sarcomas . 190
Rubinstein, L. J. Microgliomatosis 201
    Discussion 212

List of the Participants 218

Introduction

By

K. J. Zülch

Gentlemen!

I open this Symposium and bid you all a hearty welcome. The Symposium should have two objects:

1. it should clarify by scientific discussion a series of controversial problems. This is its academic significance.

2. I hope that its results will lead to an improvement of the classification of cerebral tumours and that thereby practical benefits will emerge which will help the clinician with his work and in this manner aid the sick.

First I must thank the Deutsche Forschungsgemeinschaft and the World Federation of Neurology which have supported the preparations of the Symposium financially. I would like also to thank the Springer-Verlag, Wien, which has promised to provide publication of our proceedings. It is envisaged that the present group will be established as a working commission for Neuro-Oncology within the World Federation. In this way the contact that is being made will be preserved for the future and further fruitful collaboration will be made possible.

Next I would like to welcome the participants who have agreed to contribute reports to the discussion. First of all I would like to welcome Professor *Hamperl,* Bonn, Chairman of the Nomenclature Commission of the International Union against Cancer who has kindly agreed to provide the introduction to our Symposium. I have been particularly anxious that this Symposium should achieve practical results. One I have already mentioned, I would now like to mention another: I hope that the classification which we shall have worked out will be of value to the International Union against Cancer as a basis for their further endeavours to achieve a uniform international classification. I am very happy that Professor *Hamperl* should also as a general pathologist participate in our discussion. It has always seemed important to me that we should not loose contact with our alma mater and that our discussion should always

remain within the frame work of general cancerology. I am therefore most happy that you have joined us. May I then welcome

Dr. *J. M. Brucher* (Louvain),   Dr. *M. G. Netsky* (Winston-Salem),
Dr. *W. Calvo* (Valencia),   Dr. *N. Ringertz* (Stockholm),
Dr. *G. Kersting* (München),   Dr. *L. Rubinstein* (New York),
Dr. *G. Koch* (Münster),   Dr. *G. P. Sayre* (Rochester),
Dr. *H. Luginbühl* (Bern),   Dr. *B. Schiefer* (München),
Dr. *W. Müller* (Köln),   Dr. *A. L. Woolf* (Smethwick).

The Classification of Brain Tumours

By

K. J. Zülch

Before introducing the first speaker may I say a few words of introduction to our subject. I stressed at the beginning that I hoped our discussion would not remain academic but would achieve a practical importance. Of course academic discussion is interesting, inspiring and also important. But those who have worked in close collaboration with neurosurgeons or are actually themselves clinicians feel constantly the need to make their results of value at the bedside. Of what value is the best and most enlightened classification if it has no biological significance, that is if it is not helpful to the clinician in his daily treatment of patients with tumours? We must therefore also take into account the view point of the neurosurgeon at the bedside and I believe this was the special value of the Bailey-Cushing work, that it was formed by the fusion of work carried out in collaboration by the laboratory and the clinic. This approach should and must also underline our own efforts: The survival period for successfully operated patients is the final test as to the correctness of our classification. And it is by this criterion that our classification should be orientated. A purely morphological classification may be absolutely correct from the theoretical angle but if it has no biological significance i. e. if it does not throw light on the prognosis it is for us of little value. But I believe we are all agreed on this and I need not argue the point.

I think I should however enlarge on one point and would like to make a short digression on the history of the classification of brain tumours. It seems to me that the following rule is of the greatest importance: When *Bailey* and *Cushing** published their classification, they particularly stressed the demonstration of the most frequently occuring cell types by different methods and particularly by impregnation. By comparison with the cytogenetic stages of maturation they produced a series of groups of apparently mature or immature gliomas in accordance with which the tumour material could be quite comprehensively classified. The number of unclassified cases was small and varied around 5%. They called this a histogenetic classification, although according to their first book it was a pure cytogenetic classification. If one reads the papers of

---

* See: *Bailey, P.,* and *H. Cushing,* A classification of the glioma group on a histogenetic basis with a correlated study of prognosis. Lippincott, London, 1926. — *Bailey, P.,* and *H. Cushing,* Die Gewebsverschiedenheit der Gliome und ihre Bedeutung für die Prognose. Fischer-Verlag, Jena, 1930.

1*

Bailey which followed there can be no doubting that it was in fact a histogenetic description, because in all his works you will find that he has not been predominantly concerned with descriptions of cells, but with the architecture, with the stroma and with the degenerative changes, in short with all that could be seen in the tumour tissue. This view point has in many schools remained in the background and I believe that it has been the weakness of the Hortega school: Hortega himself dwelled — as *Bailey* first did in his book with *Cushing* — predominantly on the cell type and based his classification on the individual cell. He arrived in this way at a grouping which was far removed from the actual overall morphological picture and which often had no bearing on the biological behavior. In mitigation one should remember that he received his material from the French neurosurgeon Vincent and it was virtually impossible for him to control his classification biologically. This applied equally to his later work in South America.

In general pathology we are used to taking into account the "ensemble" of the characteristics of a tumour when we wish to classify it. We are also used in neuropathology to analyse a tissue according to its individual components and then base our diagnosis on the global picture. Thus we can tell what the cells, the axons, the myelin sheaths and the vessels have contributed to the picture and what degenerative or reparative changes have taken place in these tissue components. I would like once more to stress that it seems important to me that the diagnosis should not only be based on a characteristic of the predominant cell, but on the global picture. The glioblastoma is a particularly good example for such a survey: Here it is not the type of cell, whether it will be round or spindle shaped or polymorphous which is important because these we find in many tumours. What is decisive is the overall picture, i. e. the cellularity, the number of mitoses, the tendency to growth, the degenerative changes, particularly the tendency to necrosis, the participation of the stroma in the form of the pathological vessel changes which we know so well and also the reaction of the stroma and the degenerative processes which give rise to the variegated appearon on the basis of which we make our diagnosis of a multiform glioblastoma.

I will not deny that the nature of definite cells can play an important part in the classification. I even believe that I could lead you in a — considering what I have said — almost paradoxical manner in the course of our Symposium when it comes to the classification of definitely polymorphous oligodendrogliomas. Then I may come back to this point. But I believe we have had enough theoretical introduction and I will now ask our first contributor to speak.

I. Classification of Brain Tumours
a) General Remarks on Classification

The Nomenclature of Tumours of the Nervous System

By

H. Hamperl

It has always been clear that the histological types of tumour in man remain the same whatever the epoch and whatever the region. Definite differences affect at the most the incidence — and the name. However, in order to establish differences in the incidence of tumours, it is important to agree on generally recognized names, i. e. a nomenclature which permits a comparison and thereby definite establishment of regional and temporal differences. The International Union against Cancer (UICC) has accordingly undertaken this task and already between the two world wars a Committee of experts was dedicated to this end. The work of the Committee was interrupted through the second world war and was again resumed in 1950. Since 1954 I have had the honour to be the Chairman of this Committee of the UICC which is composed of 8 scientists from all parts of the world. As a result of experience acquired in the numerous meetings of this body one became convinced that a common histological nomenclature of tumours of the brain could be of value *.

Firstly all the members of the Committee were amazed at the extent to which the nomenclatures in use at the time differed from one another. This applied not only to the different language groups, but also within a language group to the schools existing at the time. Historical development, the dominating effect of one personality, and similar factors can be reflected during long periods locally in a nomenclature, which, however, outside a particular circle, if not incomprehensible will in the final analysis appear ungrounded.

To alter such national and local peculiarities as it were by decree from above is a heavy and thankless task, because each circle is ultimately persuaded of the rightness of the name it has introduced. One must therefore often content oneself with bracketing together the designations in use in so far as they concern one and the same

---

* See: Unio Internationalis Contra Cancrum: Histological Nomenclature of Human Tumors. "Acta", Vol. XIV, 1958. — Histologische Nomenklatur menschlicher Tumoren. Zschr. Krebsforsch. *63* (1959), 75—98.

tumour type and in this way obtain a better understanding. In this way it is to be hoped that the list of synonyms will in time become narrowed in favour of a single generally accepted name.

It can immediately be appreciated that there can scarcely be any doubt that a classification introduced in the USA will already have the greatest possibility of general acceptance because the excellently edited and cheap American journals have the greatest circulation throughout the world. We should however not hold back from holding fast to another classification if we have used it previously and find it more correct than the American, a view point that our American colleagues have always recognized.

With the passage of time outstanding investigators have put forward for many pathological tumour types names which from their point of view are completely correct but have the disadvantage that they have not become accepted into the language of the country concerned. Under these circumstances nothing remains but to reject such a name. When, however, can one assume that a name has become naturalized? We believe that this is actually the case if such a name becomes taken over in a large collected work or text book — mere recognition of the name by one or another investigator in a communication to a scientific journal does not therefore satisfy us.

The volumes of the tumour atlas produced by the Armed Forces Institute of Pathology, Washington 25, D. C. have been particularly valuable in the creation of a common tumour nomenclature because one can use the excellent microscopical pictures as an aid to understanding, in that one can be persuaded of the similar significance of terms from different classifications where a picture is available. In this respect one must mention the handbook monographs of *Zülch* * and *Henschen* **.

In general, agreement can be easily obtained as to the significance of a classification if it concerns tumours which occur frequently; difficulties appear principally in regard to rare tumours concerning which the individual investigators possess only a small experience. Here it has sometimes been impossible to obtain agreement so that it is better to leave the final clarification and naming to the future, rather than establish now a name likely to be the subject of criticism.

---

* See: *Zülch, K. J.*, Biologie u. Pathologie d. Hirngeschwülste. Hdb. Neurochir., Bd. III, S. 1—702, Springer-Verlag, 1956.

** See: *Henschen, F.*, Tumoren d. Zentralnervensystems u. seiner Hüllen. Hdb. spez. path. Anat. u. Histol. Bd. XIII, Teil 3, p. 438—1040, Springer, Berlin, 1955.

IV. Tumors of nerve tissues and associated structures [1].

1. Nerve cells

Ganglioneuroma ⎫
Gangliocytoma ⎬
Ganglioglioma ⎭
Ganglioneuroblastoma ⎫⎫
Malignant ganglioneuroma ⎬⎪
Malignant gangliocytoma ⎭⎪
Malignant ganglioglioma ⎪
Sympathicogonioma
Sympathicoblastoma ⎫
Neuroblastoma ⎭

2. Neuroepithelium

Ependymoma
   epithelial
   papillary
   cellular
Malignant ependymoma ⎫
Ependymoblastoma ⎭
Papilloma of choroid plexus ⎫
Plexuspapilloma ⎭
Olfactory neuroepithelioma

3. Eye

Medulloepithelioma of ciliary ⎫
epithelium ⎬
Diktyoma ⎭
Neuroepithelioma ⎫
Retinoblastoma ⎭
   with true rosettes
   without true rosettes

4. Glia

Astrocytoma
   fibrillary
   protoplasmatic
   gemistocytic
Astrocytoma of the nose ⎫
Nasal glioma ⎭
Oligodendroglioma
Multiform glioblastoma
Polar spongioblastoma
Medulloblastoma

5. Peripheral and cranial nerves

Neurinoma ⎫
Neurilemoma ⎬
Schwannoma ⎭
Neurofibroma *
Malignant Neurinoma ⎫
Malignant Schwannoma ⎬
Malignant Neurilemoma ⎭

6. Meninges

Meningioma
   epithelioid
   meningotheliomatous ⎫
   endotheliomatous ⎭
   fibroblastic ⎫
   fibromatous ⎭
   psammomatous

7. Vascular structures of central nervous system

Haemangioma of cerebellum ⎫
   v. Hippel-Lindau's disease ⎭

8. Paraganglia

Non-chromaffin paraganglioma, ⎫
   includ. ⎪
Carotid body tumor ⎬
Glomus caroticum tumor ⎪
Chemodectoma ⎭
   adenomatoid
   angiomatoid

P. S. Some of the very rare and therefore controversial tumors and terms have not been included such as "astroblastoma", "malignant meningioma", "malignant plexus papilloma", "monstrocellular sarcoma" etc.

---

* For sarcomas arising from neurofibromas see V/1.

[1] Copied from Pamphlet of the UICC.

From this point of view the commission of the UICC seeks to devise a histological tumour nomenclature which can serve as a means of understanding between the individual investigators and language groups. In this nomenclature are naturally included the tumours of the nervous system. It lies before you in a form modified after consultation with Professor *Zülch* and it is there only as a basis for your discussion. It is of course natural that the proposed classification as well as the individual names will not satisfy any completely. Each will find defects in one place or another. One should however consider a classification as a compromise that must also be acceptable for all members of the Committee of the UICC.

I would ask you to bear in mind a few general points in relation to any considerations and objections: the whole medical nomenclature is full of classifications, which have arisen from a particular interpretation of a phenomenon. Only too frequently it has later been demonstrated that the interpretation was false when the true nature of the phenomenon became recognised. To the phenomenon however the name with its incorrect implication remained attached. As a classical example we may cite the hypernephroma which we know today without any doubt is not a suprarenal but a renal tumour. I would like therefore first to warn against changing names that have already been introduced simply because we know their basis to be incorrect. Who can guarantee that our own interpretation on which we wish to base the new name will be so correct that it will not be again deemed unsatisfactory by future generations so that a further change of name will again be necessary? If we however all designate the same phenomenon with the same name and the same term we will then have attained the object of every linguistic understanding though we should not light-heartedly introduce new names upon the scene.

The remarks just made apply above all to the repeated histogenetic approaches to the tumours of the nervous system which lie at the basis of the classification brought forward many times by *Bailey*. If we all for example envisage by medulloblastoma the same type of tumour, then I see no obvious and pressing need to change the name even if the origin of these tumours from medulloblasts is doubtful.

It is very common to apply to the tumours of the nervous system the suffix "blastoma", which usually implies that the tumour cells correspond to the formative cells at a certain stage of embryonic development. Basically the use of the term does not imply that we are dealing with a particularly malignant tumour though, of course, because of their embryonic immaturity many tumours are actually of an extremely malignant nature.

As with many other tumours there occur amongst the tumours of the nervous system all stages between outspokenly benign tumours up to those bringing about the end of the life of the patient in the shortest time and therefore to be considered of the highest malignancy. One seeks to draw attention to these "grades of malignancy" — which have previously been discussed by *Virchow* and particularly by my teacher *Rössle** in different ways. Thus for example the grading system inaugurated by *Broders* and the *Mayo* Clinic has been extended to the tumours of the nervous system in that in many tumours four different grades are distinguished. The European pathologists and neuropathologists follow very hesitatingly, if at all, this system; they incline much more to the view that the tumours belonging to the individual grades in malignancy should be regarded as particular types with particular names or they indicate them by an adjective as a sub-group of one and the same tumour.

The Committee of the UICC will be glad to take up any suggestion coming from this special meeting and seek to obtain for you the appropriate recognition if it is in any way reconcilable with the basic principles which I have indicated in my introduction as binding for the work of the Commission.

Discussion

Dr. Zülch: Thank you so much, Dr. Hamperl, for your clear and I think very useful discussion which will be of great value in giving our discussions a sense of direction. All symposia are liable to lose sight of their objective and I think you have given us a straight line which the first morning's discussions may now follow. Will you open your suggestion to discussion?

Dr. Hamperl: Yes.

Dr. Netsky: Dr. Hamperl, the term malignancy for me has clinical as well as histologic implications. Would it not be better to use the term poorly differentiated rather than malignant? Poor differentiation can be seen in slides, but not clinical malignancy.

Dr. Hamperl: Yes, you are just starting at the top. So, you see, there are different numbers 1 to 8 in our classification which concern the structures from which the tumours are derived. This follows the pattern set by the committee. The first group concerns the nerve cells and we decided to refer here to the tumours which are derived from the normal ganglion or neuron cells as ganglioneuroma or gangliocytoma in the case of the benign ones and

---

* See: *Rössle, R.,* Stufen der Malignität. Sitzungsber. d. Dtsch. Akademie d. Wissenschaften, Berlin, 1949. Akademie-Verlag. Berlin, 1950.

ganglioneuroblastoma for the malignant ones, the term blastoma usually meaning that the tumour is more immature and malignant. As synonyms we suggest malignant ganglioneuroma and malignant gangliocytoma. I was told that these expressions are in use so what you say could only be an addition. Do you use the name?

Dr. Netsky: I use it and I think it is better because as I say it is what one sees. One does not see clinical malignancy in a slide, but rather the degree of differentiation.

Dr. Zülch: Don't you see malignancy? I think perhaps we can make the problem a little bit clearer if we accept that there are two aspects of malignancy as you have already implied. There is clinical malignancy and malignancy of growth. This is particularly true for the skull, because the skull is one of the body cavities which is rigid and a histologically very benign tumour may be clinically highly malignant, an astrocytoma of the frontal lobe will only endanger life after three, four, five years, while an astrocytoma of the aqueduct may be fatal in the first year. So I think we have to differentiate two forms of malignancy and perhaps you as a general pathologist would like to give us the definition of malignancy of growth.

Dr. Hamperl: Malignancy can be due to a rapid growth which is always combined with destruction. Or malignancy can be based on the special localisation. A benign tumour occluding the aqueduct may kill a man, a benign island cell tumour of the pancreas may also by its production of insulin kill a man, but the pathologist would see a benign island cell tumour. So it is a very controversial matter, almost philosophical and I would rather not discuss it too extensively here because I fear the French will say as they said once when the Germans discussed the implications of inflammation, c'est une question allemande!

Dr. Rubinstein: If we are going to examine systematically, Dr. Hamperl, the classification and nomenclature of tumours, we must seek agreement on the existence of clinical and pathological entities. Now starting with the first list of tumours there is not even as far as I am aware agreement as to the existence of some of the entities described here. Some people deny the existence of ganglio-neuroma and gangliocytoma in the CNS. This is a point that needs to be established, before we can even start on the nomenclature.

Dr. Hamperl: Yes, that some people say it does not exist or some people say we should call it something else does not abolish the fact that these names are used by some people and even used as legends for pictures. So if Willis and others would not like to use this word they should say what they would term this picture.

Dr. Rubinstein: I think it is regarded by some as a hamartoma. I think, Dr. Netsky perhaps would agree with this.

Dr. Hamperl: Yes, let's finish the discussion about it.

Dr. Zülch: Yes, I think these are hamartomas with autonomous growth. So I would say this is only a special form of a blastoma, Dr. Netsky, I think, agrees on this.

Dr. Rubinstein: Indeed I was going to suggest to-morrow that these tumours, the ganglioneuromas of the CNS, very frequently show an astrocytic element and the malignant features of the tumour depend largely on the astrocytic element. This is in accordance with the other term used by Courville: ganglio-glioma. And important implications for the spread and biological behaviour of the tumour.

Dr. Hamperl: I am quite willing to include as synonyms here terms suggested by you if they are used by a reasonably wide circle of neurosurgeons.

Dr. Zülch: Our whole aim can only be a compromise, because we are gathered here like the United Nations and have got to make a resolution at the end, that means we have to mute to some extent our personal feelings. You know that the classification before you is not my personal classification but I have accepted many items so as to get a compromise which is acceptable.

Dr. Hamperl: I am quite willing to change my terms if you tell me that the specialists use the term ganglioglioma and mean by this a tumour which other people call a ganglioneuroma or gangliocytoma.

Dr. Zülch: Then we can say malignant ganglioglioma. That is alright then. We will have both entities. Dr. Ringertz?

Dr. Ringertz: But of these three groups here I would only take one name from each: ganglioneuroma, ganglioneuroblastoma and sympathicoblastoma. These tumours are very well known in the sympathetic tract, not in the central nervous system. And they are all neural in origin. So if we should put in ganglioglioma I would propose that it should be taken as a quite separate group, not as a synonym to ganglioneuroma: a) ganglioglioma, b) ganglioneuroma, c) ganglioneuroblastoma and d) sympathicoblastoma. — Another question: We are perhaps coming to this but I should like to know what is the difference between sympathicogonioma and sympathicoblastoma, because I am not aware of any.

Dr. Hamperl: Yes, I agree with you, I am not an expert in this kind of tumour but in suggesting an alteration I would always appreciate an illustration to what has been suggested in a generally recognized atlas, text book or hand-book.

Dr. Ringertz: Dr. Zülch's excellent book, for example, you have accepted the term ganglioglioma haven't you?

Dr. Zülch: No, I discussed it, but I preferred gangliocytoma and qualifying it as in Germany we very often do according to the neuropathological school of Bielschowsky and the men who followed him, by adding a second adjective to characterize it, like — amyelinic, myelinic, glial and so on.

But I should like to hear Dr. Kersting's remark on this, because he made a very penetrating remark, he said, this discussion on the classification ought to take place on the 3rd day of our Symposium. I take his point but I think it ought not to take place the 3rd day but in 3, or 5 or 10 years, after we have discussed all these tumour groups in detail and have come to a conclusion, if we ever come to any. So, please, do consider this discussion as aimed at obtaining a compromise, if we cannot solve the theoretical problems, at least we may perhaps diminish the "Unschönheiten" of this nomenclature, and help Dr. Hamperl to prepare a classification which he can present to his commission. Nobody will be bound to the new classification as the South American neuropathologists felt they were to Hortaga, as he was dying, to adopt his classification. There is no such obligation here. It may be a help to have the synonyms grouped. I would not project here a table of the synonyms of 3 or 4 groups. I may do that tomorrow, I mean you know all that and you all will be astounded to see the various varieties. So I think to come to a practical consequence of our discussion, I would make another suggestion, that anybody who wishes to make a further contribution to the discussion after he has returned home may send it either to you or to me and I will make a digest and we can go over the matter again.

Dr. Hamperl: That is, in my opinion, a very good suggestion as to the procedure. Now your remark about the undifferentiated tumours.

Dr. Zülch: I think that I am following your line of thought. The malignancy of tumours has always-been the subject of discussion to us. I think, if you estimate the number of mitoses and the cell structure of a medulloblastoma and then do the same with an oligodendroglioma and assess their malignancy from the general pathological stand point but without knowledge of the biological significance of these two tumours, you will judge both of them to be equally malignant. Yet the medulloblastoma will kill the patient in 8 months, while a patient with an oligodendroglioma may survive 3 or 4 years. The malignancy of some tumours, and I expect you will agree with this, can only be assessed by their biological behaviour, that is by postoperative survival period. This has been the practice for a long time already. Thus Lebert in 1851 reported the first study of the malignancy of brain tumours, and based it on the survival period of patients. On the other hand there are reliable histological signs of malignancy. For instance in comparing a glioblastoma with an astrocytoma, we are influenced by the number of necroses, the unorderly form of the stroma, the size of the vessels, the number of mitoses and so many other characteristics, all of which give a hint of the malignancy of the glioblastoma, though we could not easily define the theoretical basis for our conclusion. So I should rather be in favour of retaining the term malignant instead of poorly differentiated.

Dr. Hamperl: I think it was most unfortunate that we started with the first group of tumours which happened to be a rare one. I would prefer to proceed to a less debateable one but first I would answer the question by Dr. Ringertz about sympathogonioma and sympathicoblastoma. This was included by the wish of the late Prof. Oberling, as he, as a pupil of Masson used to make this differentiation. In the text-book of Masson you will find two very good illustrations and even in the fascicle of Kernohan *, or possibly, Karsner's fascicle *, you will find two different pictures, one labelled sympathicogonioma and the other sympathicoblastoma. We could not do otherwise than include both types of tumours, but I personally feel that there is a difference though we cannot perceive it in every case.

Dr. Zülch: Dr. Rubinstein, you wanted to say something, I see.

Dr. Rubinstein: Two tumours, the malignant ganglioneuroma and the malignant gangliocytoma are listed here. Now, how do you recognize a malignant ganglioneuroma or a malignant gangliocytoma, as both are fully differentiated? From my own experience I am unable to recognize either of them. Once these tumour cells do become malignant, as they very rarely do, they lose their neuronal characteristics.

Dr. Zülch: May I object. I could show you a gangliocytoma with fully differentiated ganglion cells with Nissl bodies, but full of mitoses and with a survival period of only 6 to 8 months. So this is definitely a malignant gangliocytoma or -neuroma.

Dr. Rubinstein: I have cases like that too, Dr. Zülch. You see, I am not sure whether the cells we call malignant because of their mitoses are actually neurones.

Dr. Zülch: Well, mine are definitely neurones if you can recognize cells at all. You think that the smaller cells or the cells which undergo mitosis are not neurones?

Dr. Rubinstein: Is there any evidence that they are?

Dr. Zülch: Well, 80% of the tumour consists of ganglion cells and the rest of mitotic and lymphoid cells. I know that you are hinting at the mixed tumours

---

* Armed Forces Institute of Pathology, Washington 25, D. C., fascicles 35 and 37, *Kernohan, J. W.,* and *G. P. Sayre,* Tumors of the central nervous system (1952), resp. fasc. 29, *Karsner, H. T.,* Tumors of the adrenal (1950).

again, but in this case I am pretty convinced that even ganglion cells may be malignant enough to divide by mitotic activity. They do that during maturation, don't they? The germinal layer is full of mitoses of ganglion cells. Is that correct? Why should they not regress back to the primitive stage? That is very often seen in general pathology.

Dr. Rubinstein: That's still a question of cytological interpretation, and I would not absolutely deny the possibility, Dr. Zülch. But I think it is very difficult to be absolutely convinced this is so. My point of view may be based particularly on a case of ganglion cell tumour where as far as I can see the malignancy is entirely confined to the glial element. I know the case that you described the pictures, I agree, are convincing.

(Hdbch. d. Neurochir. Bd. III, Abb. 274.)

Dr. Zülch: Well, could we not meet this difficulty by saying malignant ganglioglioma, and then we have the ganglion and the gliomatous part in it, and Dr. Hamperl, I am sure, will...

Dr. Hamperl, Yes, I do. Now I have to point out to you that we had in our original draft medulloblastoma here as the next entity. But Dr. Zülch advises me that the medulloblastoma should be better listed in the group 4 glia. So we took it out here because the derivation from nerve cells of the medulloblastoma is more than doubtful. We may discuss this later.

Dr. Kersting: That is against the demonstration by Dr. Lumsden using tissue culture but agrees with my findings. There were two differences between us as Dr. Lumsden showed neurites proliferating in cultures of medulloblastoma. We showed that neurites neither exist in our cultures of medulloblastoma or those of neuro-epitheliomas or retinoblastomas (12 cultures of medulloblastoma and 12 of retinoblastomas) *.

Dr. Rubinstein: The medulloblastomas are a vast group in which some differentiate towards glial elements and other neurons and I think, it is very interesting that you have this complementary evidence to Lumsden's.

Dr. Zülch: Would you proceed now, Dr. Hamperl?

Dr. Hamperl: We proceed now to group 2, which we should call neuro-epithial. You see, there are only two kinds of ependymoma, ependymoma and malignant ependymoma or ependymoblastoma. And the benign one is sub-divided in epithelial, papillary and cellular and they are demonstrated by the appropriate pictures in Kernohan's fascicle and the last one here is papilloma of the choroid plexus. We eliminated from here on Dr. Zülch's suggestion the olfactory neuroepithelioma which we put near the nasal glioma and a tumour which Oberling insisted upon as esthesio-neuroepithelioma.

Dr. Rubinstein: I wonder if I may add a point about the olfactory tumours. We accepted these very rare tumours, as one form of peripheral neuroblastomas, the olfactory neuroblastomas. I think they are different from the nasal gliomas which are composed of much more mature cells. I think we have two different tumours here, the nasal glioma which is a congenital tumour occuring in children and consisting mainly of astrocytes and then there is a very charac-teristic tumour arising in the nasal fossa which is almost indistinguishable from sympathicoblastoma.

Dr. Ringertz: I entirely agree with two kinds of nasal glioma, one kind is a tumour rather like the medulloblastoma of the cerebellum and the neuro-blastomas of the peripheral nervous system and the other one is a much more differentiated glial tumour.

---

* See: *Kersting, G.,* Die Gewebszüchtung menschlicher Hirngeschwülste, Springer-Verlag, Berlin-Göttingen-Heidelberg, 1961.

Dr. Zülch: How common are these? I have never seen one.

Unidentified: They are very rare.

Dr. Zülch: Well, do we need to include these in our classification, because, if I would follow this line, I could add at least ten different entities and if I go to Dr. Hallervorden's collection I may find another twenty. By the way Dr. Schiefer will be able to show us a very good example of this nasal malignant tumour at the night session today. But do we need to introduce it into this general classification? Does anyone think we need it for practical purposes? Because we don't want to include rarities ...

Dr. Sayre: I would imagine that it would be of value for the classification to have a section 9 in which to group the rare tumours. Then people using the classification will realize that in addition to the 8 major variants there is a whole series of tumours of questionable etiology and questionable terminology. They should be listed separately.

Dr. Zülch: I think this is a good suggestion.

Dr. Hamperl: I will have to make a note. Not of a 9th group but a note that in spite of all these subdivisions there are tumours that do not fit in here and which are listed separately.

Dr. Müller: I think the malignant plexus papilloma also belongs to this last group of very rare tumours.

Dr. Zülch: There are indeed very rare cases of malignant transformation.

Dr. Hamperl: I have never seen one personally and I have not seen a picture in Kernohan's book.

Dr. Zülch: No, but we have published one, Dr. Müller * has 2, and we know they definitely occur (van Hoytema) **

Dr. Ringertz: I have one, too.

Dr. Hamperl: I accept it. But if we put in the classification every kind of tumour that has been published at one time or another, it will swell up, and the man who would like to use this — a pathologist far in the desert — will not be able to do so. — Let us proceed then. We come to the neuroepithelioma and on a suggestion of Dr. Zülch we made a distinction between one with true rosettes and one without true rosettes.

Dr. Zülch: We have forgotten the term retinoblastoma, we need to add it because it is the most common name.

Dr. Hamperl: I think this suggestion is very good, otherwise people who do not find rosettes will say it is not a neuroepithelioma or a retinoblastoma. We have to put in two pictures, one with rosettes and the other one without.

Dr. Zülch: Yes, and both in fact occur.

Dr. Hamperl: Finally the malignant melanoma of the uveal tract should be added. — Now we proceed to a group where most of the brain tumours are included and we have first the astrocytoma, as you see, with various subgroups. On a suggestion of Dr. Zülch we left out the term astroblastoma. And now I would like to hear your opinion. Is astroblastoma used sometimes or not?

Dr. Ringertz: Naturally astroblastoma has been defined and there is histologically such a type of tumour, but if we are to have a classification for practical purposes I would propose that it should be left out, because most of these astroblastomas fall into the group where we have the gemistocytic astrocytomas.

Dr. Hamperl: Yes, this is my opinion too.

---

* *Müller:* see *Cardauns, H.,* Über ein malignes Plexuspapillom, Zbl. Neurochir. *17* (1957), 349—353.

** *Van Hoytema, G. J.,* and *W. E. Winckel,* Zur Frage des primären Plexuskarzinoms, Zbl. Neurochir. *17* (1957), 353—363.

Dr. Kersting: I am of the opinion that astroblastomas definitely do exist. They are very rare — I have only one in our series but there are certain characteristics. You find the tumour in young people. And *in vitro* it shows a cycle of development which I may perhaps show you ...

Dr. Rubinstein: I would like to support Dr. Kersting on this. I think the astroblastomas do exist as a pathological entity though they are excessively rare as Dr. Kersting says. I have only seen four cases myself. The problem of course has been put forward by Bayley who included a number of these in his original paper and I am certain that some of these are sufficiently malignant to constitute glioblastomas, Dr. Zülch * has discussed this question and included the astroblastoma among the astrocytomas. There is, I think, a point I would like to emphasize that is relevant to Dr. Ringertz's point of view regarding the relationship with the gemistocytic astrocytoma. The gemistocytic astrocytomas very often show a perivascular structure, but this does not make them astroblastomas. The astroblastoma is very characteristic and is not composed of typical gemistocytic cells. It is an almost pure tumour, and is composed entirely of cells arranged around blood vessels with fine processes towards them.

Dr. Zülch: I agree completely with all of you, that there is a rare form of astrocytic tumour which corresponds to Bailey's original astroblastoma. The reason why I suggested omitting it was that the Hortega school has a completely different definition of astroblastoma. To get rid of this confusion and the misunderstanding between the South Americans and ourselves, I suggested leaving it out, but we could have a compromise and to this end I would put forward for discussion a fourth group of astrocytomas — astroblastic astrocytoma. Then everybody will understand that this is an astrocytoma in which astroblastic formations are very common, because as you correctly said, Dr. Rubinstein, in the original paper of Bailey there were some glioblastomas with astroblasts and there were also astrocytomas with astroblasts, and this made the confussion complete. Perhaps we can say astroblastic astrocytoma and thereby get rid of this confusion in the long run.

Dr. Luginbühl: I would like to make a linguistic remark. I think, the term gemistocytic is a very inappropriate expression, a horrible word. We should not mix up English and German language in such a horrible way.

Dr. Rubinstein: γεμιζειν means to stuff in Greek, it is a perfectly good term.

Dr. Zülch: May I ask in the meantime Dr. Woolf to repeat one suggestion he made yesterday. He felt in looking through this classification, the need to underline those names which we think are most desirable and leave the synonyms unstressed. This could be done without hurting other authors' feelings too much. I think even if it strikes every one of us who has suggested something, we would all agree that those which are considered most useful or best ought to be underlined or marked in some way. Perhaps you would like to comment on that yourself, Dr. Woolf.

Dr. Woolf: Yes, that's quite right, I did say that, because I think 90% of human beings never read accompanying instructions. They look at a list like this and they get the impression that each of these names refers to a different tumour, they don't realize they are synonyms and I hope I am not insulting general pathologists when I think that many of them will look at this long list and say "well, that confirms me in my impression that cerebral tumours are too difficult for me even to try to study." I do think it would be a good thing if somehow the situation could be simplified. If it is not possible to shorten the

---

* See *Zülch, K. J.,* Das Glioblastom, morphologisch und biologisch gesehen. Acta Neurochir. Suppl. VI (1959), 1—30.

list and it does seem as if we were adding to it more than we are subtracting
from it in the version we are recommending to the Union, perhaps we could
in the proceedings of this meeting indicate which terms we in this meeting think
are preferable. I don't think Dr. Hamperl can very easily start emphasizing names
in this list because it implicates many other people outside this room. But we
could in a comment on the discussion, say the Symposium was in favour of these
particular synonyms — if we can agree.

Dr. Hamperl: I am completely in agreement with Dr. Luginbühl that the word
gemistocytic is a terrible one. But we should not depart from our principle which
is to put in the list all the words used in any wide circle or linguistic group. And
as this is used in the United States and has even cropped up in the "Fascicles" *
we have to keep it whatever our feelings are about it. The second remark concerns
Dr. Woolf's proposal. In fact we had in the preparing of this nomenclature
exactly followed his advice, underlined the terms we thought would suit best
and then put in brackets terms which should be avoided and, in between, terms
which could be used. But people mainly from England resented this classification
and they said we were not entitled to be judges on other people's customs. So
we decided to drop this and simply put the most suitable term on the top of the
list and trust that everybody's eye falls first on the name at the top of the list
of synonyms and that they would view the others as second and third choice.
What you were afraid of, that synonyms and entities could be confused can be
easily avoided by the printing. You see we print every term with a wide space
between each other, so the list is very easy to grasp and confusion between the
types and synonyms will not occur. It is a matter for the printer. Of course
I think it would be very nice if this conference could point out the most desired
terms and put them on top of the list of the synonyms. But I think this could be
done at the end when we have been through.

Dr. Zülch: Dr. Hamperl, would you proceed with the discussion on the glia
tumours?

Dr. Hamperl: We have suggested three subdivisions of astrocytomas: fibrillary,
protoplasmatic — we shall refer to a picture of Zülch's book — gigantocellular
or gemistocytic. We now have the questions as to whether we should add a
fourth one or if you think this is enough for the beginning.

Dr. Netsky: In view of what is known and to abbreviate this classification
may I suggest that those subtitles of astrocytomas be eliminated. I know of
no clinical justification. One can simply call it astrocytoma.

Dr. Rubinstein: To try to simplify too much a subject which is already very
complicated is I think dangerous. If simplifying means that one is going to
reject established entities, the classification is likely to fail in its purpose.

Dr. Netsky: May I ask what is the theory of this subdivision into fibrillary,
protoplasmatic and so on, what is the use?

Dr. Rubinstein: Well, the use of it is that the pathologist is faced with the
histological diagnosis. If he sees the specimen from operation he has got to make
his diagnosis on certain characteristic patterns. He has got to recognize the type
of cells he is going to visualize in order to make the diagnosis. He must be
aware of the various forms which astrocytomas may take. The problem is seen
best in regard to the meningiomas. Although it is quite useless from a practical
point of view to subdivide meningiomas into fibroblastic, meningothelial, etc.
it is important for the diagnostician to be aware of the existence of different
patterns and cell forms. That is, I think, the practical use of the histological
subdivision.

* Fascicles of the Armed Forces Institute of Pathology, Washington 25, D. C.

Dr. Netsky: The issue here is what is most useful for the pathologists throughout the world and I feel that if these subdivisions, which I think clinically and histologically are unnecessary, are continued they make the subject much more difficult than it is. I believe this view is justified since I find no particular practical or clinical use for the subdivisions of astrocytomas or even meningiomas. It is my practice to call them astrocytomas or meningiomas and that is sufficient for the clinician and for all.

Dr. Zülch: Would you like to comment on this, Dr. Hamperl?

Dr. Hamperl: What do you think about grading the astrocytomas into four grades?

Dr. Sayre: Of course the problem of the grading of tumour is one which occupies a place in the later discussion of this meeting when I hope I will be able to persuade some of the people who don't like grading that it has its values; I think it is too early at the present time, we will never get through our morning's discussion if we discuss the subject in detail now. I do hope that Dr. Hamperl will keep his classification open however for further discussion on this matter. Dr. Hamperl has pointed out several times that the classification in use is based upon descriptions which have been published and which are in use and for that reason, I think, the question of grading is one which must be discussed before a final draft is prepared.

Dr. Zülch: Would you kindly proceed, Dr. Hamperl.

Dr. Hamperl: Yes, I have taken a note that some members of the group here think that we could leave out the subgroups of astrocytomas, whereas others think that subgroups may be a help for classifying this rather large group of tumours.

Dr. Zülch: Well, may I then suggest just in order to get rid of the South American definition of astroblastoma which is hopelessly undefined that we create a fourth group of astroblastic astrocytomas. So long as these 4 groups exist it will make clear that there is a subdivision of astrocytoma which is characterised by the occurrence of astroblasts.

Dr. Hamperl: Let us consider the proposition of Dr. Zülch that we put in an astroblastoma. Should we put it in as a special group or as astroblastic astrocytoma. I think astroblastoma has been used as a special group of tumour.

Dr. Kersting: But in a different sense. The astroblastomas of Hortega are mainly ependymomas.

Dr. Zülch: Not only ependymomas. He includes everything in it.

Dr. Rubinstein: I wonder if I can make a suggestion here for our further work. Perhaps we can leave on one side these very rare tumours — we agree they are, like the ganglion cell tumours very rare — and may I suggest a practical proposition that some sort of tumour registry is organised, to which rare tumours can be sent so that finally a large collection can be established to decide whether these entities do exist from the practical point of view. Perhaps this can be revised every few years. I think the astroblastoma is a case in point. Once you get a collection of 10 or 15 cases gathered from all over the world, you can come to a conclusion whether they do exist as a separate entity or not.

Dr. Zülch: Thank you very much, Dr. Rubinstein, I think that the World Federation of Neurology would be very much in favour of this. They have promised to have a standing study group with a secretary who ought to prepare further meetings and they are, also in favour of a collection of examples. They suggested having the secretary of the group here in Cologne. This is *, of course, still open to discussion, but Dr. van Bogaert made this suggestion and we have already made a start with the tumour collection of the German Society of Neuro-surgeons and I think that the specimens which you have sent in here for discussion may be a further very valuable and appreciated addition to this collection. So we could start here such a registry and opportunity to study the collection will be given to everybody who wishes it.

Dr. Hamperl: Going back to our previous discussion I take it, that you, Dr. Rubinstein, think the case of the astroblastoma is not too clear yet and it is better to leave it out as it is a very rare tumour.

Dr. Calvo: I would like to make a comment about the morphology of the astroblasts. The form of the astroblast when impregnated by the silver carbonate method of Hortega or the silver oxide methode of Cajal can be simulated by cells of various origins. For example: We may see cells that look like an astroblast in a gemistocytic astrocytoma. Even a reactive astrocyte can look like an astroblast, because when the cell is dying it loses first the expansions that are opposite to the blood vessel while the expansions of the cell which form the vascular feet are enlarged so that it looks like an astroblast. We could distinguish these cells from an astroblast, because there are nuclei without a membrane, usually opposite the vascular feet. Another way in which cells are produced looking like astroblasts is seen in rapidly growing astrocytomas. These are cells that have no time to develop all their expansions because they divide so quickly. These cells are mixed with other types of cells in glioblastomas. We should not classify these tumours as astroblastomas because we find a few cells looking like astroblasts. I never saw a tumour that looked like a pure astroblastoma. It was always related to an ependymoma of cellular type in which the slowly growing cells have time to develop opposite to the vascular feet a few short expansions that even divided in a little tree opposite the blood vessel. So if we envisage a pure form of astroblastoma, this form I think should be related to the ependymomas of more mature type.

Dr. Zülch: I think, this valuable contribution from our critical friend of the Hortega school suggests that we should leave out the astroblastomas all together and now we can go on with our practical work. Dr. Hamperl, would you comment on the next group.

Dr. Hamperl: The further groups are: oligodendroglioma, malignant oligo-dendroglioma with a picture from Zülch, multiform glioblastoma, polar spongio-blastoma and at last medulloblastoma here.

Then we proceed to group 5: Peripheral nerves. There are three synonyms listed: Neurinoma, Neurolemmoma and schwannoma. It is very difficult to know which one to favour. In America I think Neurolemmoma or schwannoma is in use.

Dr. Zülch: Acoustic neurinoma is very common at least with the neuro-surgeons.

Dr. Hamperl: Everybody will accept neurofibroma, and as well malignant neurinoma, Neurolemmoma and schwannoma, as the malignant counterpart.

Dr. Rubinstein: The question of malignancy here is important as there are surely cases of neurofibroma which become malignant. And these should be regarded as neurofibrosarcomas. I think that these are different from the malignant schwannoma. If you accept there is a difference between a schwannoma or Neurolemmoma on one hand and neurofibroma on the other, similarly I think

Problem Commission for Neurooncology Secretary: Prof. Dr. *K. J. Zülch,* Städt. Krankenanstalt, Ostmerheimer Straße 200, Köln, Deutschland.

the malignant form must be differentiated. I would suggest that we add neurofibrosarcoma to the list.

Dr. Kersting: Well, I am asking whether neurofibroma has to be included in this list.

Dr. Zülch: Well, these are peripheral nerve tumours and there must be a blastoma type for Recklinghausen's disease...

Dr. Kersting: ... because it is a fibroma primarily?

Dr. Zülch: Is it?

Dr. Hamperl: We are not so convinced that it is a pure fibroma of the nerves because the Schwann cells take a very special part in its formation as Masson pointed out very distinctly. Now about the sarcoma arising from a neurofibroma. This is a not so rare occurrence because I have seen several cases on the autopsy table of patients with neurofibromatosis dying from a sarcoma. But if you would give me a section of such a sarcoma and not say that it was derived from a neurofibroma, I would not be able to make a diagnosis of malignant neurofibrosarcoma. It is just a plain sarcoma without any traces of the mother tissue from which it arose.

Dr. Rubinstein: Since neurofibroma does become malignant one cannot just eliminate it as an entity by omitting it from the classification. Don't you agree?

Dr. Hamperl: We could make a note here, that sarcomas arising from neurofibromas show the same picture as sarcomas arising from connective tissue.

Dr. Koch: I would like to ask whether there are histological differences between the unilateral and the bilateral acoustic neurinomas?

Dr. Zülch: Who would like to comment? Dr. Sayre?

Dr. Sayre: Having seen a few I would say that it is practically impossible to differentiate. I have never been successful in doing so.

Dr. Ringertz: I would like to mention that the other year I was in a Symposium like this one, but organized by the World Health Organisation, on soft tissue tumours and there it was decided that we should have a malignant neurinoma as it is quite recognizable. But we did not put in a special type called malignant neurofibroma, because we decided that this was in fact indistinguishable from an ordinary fibrosarcoma.

Dr. Hamperl: I will put in a note about sarcoma arising from neurofibromas and add: see "connective tissue", and that will deal with this matter. Thank you. Now we come to "the meninges" with the meningioma; there are several subgroups and now I have to ask you about the three subgroups: meningotheliomatous, endotheliomatous or epithelioid in the first one, fibroblastic or fibromatous is the second. In our first draft we had one which was called psammomatous, but Dr. Zülch pointed out to me that psammoma bodies are a common phenomenon of all meningiomas and should not be used to construct subgroups. Instead of this he proposed including a group of angioblastic meningiomas. What do you think about this?

Dr. Ringertz: Yes, I am quite in favour of including an angioblastic type, I know that Kernohan has eliminated it, but I don't agree with this, because there are some meningiomas which in my opinion are definitely angioblastic.

Dr. Zülch: Dr. Sayre, would you like to comment?

Dr. Sayre: Only that where there are angioblastic meningiomas there is not very much difference from angioblastomas elsewhere, and I cannot see why they should be considered as special tumours of the brain.

Dr. Zülch: Angioblastomas in the cerebellum infiltrate, angioblastic meningiomas never because they are definitely encapsulated. I think this is a definite difference, they behave different clinically. It is the only group, even in the

Cushing and Eisenhardt * book which has a worse diagnosis than the others. So I think both clinically and morphologically it is worthwhile differentiating them, if you are going to differentiate meningiomas into subgroups at all.

Dr. Sayre: Do you feel angioblastic meningiomas as a tumour behave different from the angioblastomas occuring elsewhere?

Dr. Ringertz: Yes, quite definitely.

Dr. Netsky: I should like to propose another classification, that is, human beings who are pathologists are lumpers or splitters. I am basically a lumper, and I would suggest that we lump all these varieties together. I find no practical or clinical advantage in separating them into innumerable subdivisions. They should all be called meningiomas.

Dr. Rubinstein: I would like to support Dr. Zülch on this point. The angioblastic meningioma certainly seems to have a worse prognosis than the other varieties and I think there is something to be said for being a splitter sometimes, Dr. Netsky.

Dr. Zülch: Now on clinical grounds I would support Dr. Netsky. I think Dr. Müller follows our practice, we say meningioma and we put in brackets what type it is, just for academic reasons. The clinician does not wish to know it.

Dr. Hamperl: Well, I take it that you are in favour of leaving out the psammomas. Good. For malignant meningioma, meningoblastoma, we will have pictures provided by Zülch.

With the vascular tumours we have the haemangioma of the cerebellum, we put "Lindau" in brackets, because it is the type of angioma occuring in Lindau's disease.

Furthermore Zülch has convinced me that he has had several cases of monstrocellular sarcomas which are probably originating from the vessels or the connective tissue accompanying the vessels. So I am very much in favour of putting it in here because I have myself seen it in several cases where there was always a doubt as to what kind of tumour it was.

Dr. Zülch: Dr. Kersting, would you like to comment on the tissue cultures?

Dr. Kersting: I can only support the concept of a monstrocellular sarcoma, because in tissue culture the tumour cells behave quite differently from those in gliomatous tumours such as the glioblastomas.

Dr. Zülch: Well, there is a very nice historical story with regard to this. Dr. Scherer was working at Rössle's institute on gliomas and you all know his three famous glioma studies. He was however very anti-american, as you will remember and never accepted the "American classification" which he hated and to ridicule it he said: "Well, how can you call a tumour like this a glioma or glioblastoma", (and then he depicted a typical monstrocellular sarcoma,) "when in the vertebral column we have exactly the same tumour". But he only showed that this polymorphous tumour was probably of mesodermal origin and his attack against the American classification was definitely inadequate. — Any other comment?

Dr. Rubinstein: I must comment on the monstrocellular sarcoma, because I must record here my own reservations on this entity. I would suggest perhaps since some people do not accept them that again this is a tumour which is worth studying on a registry basis so that one can accumulate a number of cases. Now we have certainly seen tumours which do correspond to what Dr. Zülch has

---

* See: *Cushing, H.,* and *L. Eisenhardt,* Meningiomas (their classification, regional behavior, life history and surgical end results). Thomas, Springfield and Baltimore, 1938.

described as monstrocellular sarcoma. But I have reservations on two counts. First we were not certain that they constitute a single entity and in some of the cases thought the diagnosis was mainly glioblastoma with very large cells, while others certainly seem to be sarcomatous. But as far as I can correlate the picture in our cases with those of Dr. Zülch our impression is that some of the perivascular sarcomas were mixed tumours and I am going to discuss this tomorrow. This is again a type of tumour which is worth considerable examination and I agree there is room for discussion.

Dr. Zülch: Thank you, Dr. Rubinstein. Dr. Calvo, would you comment on this, because in your cases is a wonderful example which in the aniline preparations you would probably diagnose as a monstrocellular sarcoma. Yet the impregnations show that is a glioblastoma. So I think we all would make a differential diagnosis between the two types on the basis of good impregnations and tissue culture of course if possible. Would you comment on this, Dr. Calvo?

Dr. Calvo: I brought with me one of these cases in which there are monster cells derived from the glial elements because of this discussion of the monstrocellular sarcoma. With the silver impregnation it is quite clear which structures are which. Whenever we see a gliovascular relationship it should be recognized that we are dealing with a glioma and whenever we see cells surrounded by nets of reticulin it must be a sarcoma. And as we have both cases here we may see a little later how easy it is to distinguish one from the other. But not on nuclear staining.

Dr. Zülch: Thank you, Dr. Calvo.

Dr. Woolf: I want to suggest that we have a synonym "giant cell sarcoma" here, because as far as I know we have never had before in England this prefix monstro- and while if everyone is agreed on monstrocellular as being the best term I am in favour of our using it, we should make a definite decision as to which term we prefer. I would suggest that giant cell may be just as good, because we are quite familiar with giant cells. I just put this forward for discussion. I hope we all emerge with only one term, whatever happens.

Dr. Hamperl: What is your opinion, Dr. Zülch?

Dr. Zülch: Well, you know that the author always fights for his own name and I thought that this name was most appropriate. Again it is very interesting historically that Schmincke was the first to demonstrate an example. He measured the cells and said they were 400 microns in diameter and indeed they are almost visible to the naked eye, which is really extraordinary in the body. Why should we not call them monsters? They are definitely cell "monsters", because they are really as Schmincke said, not comparable with any other cell in the body. So I agree with the synonym, but I still fight for the "monster".

Dr. Woolf: Is this an exceptionable term in German too, this monstrocellular, or is it a common term for giant cells?

Dr. Zülch: No, but is has been accepted by many German neurosurgeons and pathologists.

Dr. Hamperl: We have several tumours at other sites of the human body which we call giant cell tumours of the tendons and so on, but monstrocellular tumour, this is the only one where we use the name monster.

Dr. Woolf: I see, it does imply something special.

Dr. Calvo: I was going to make the same comments as Dr. Hamperl because the giant cell tumours could be confused with those of the tendons, and these are real monster cells in the sarcomas.

Dr. Ringertz: I wonder if we should not postpone the discussion about including the monstrocellular tumours with these vascular tumours, until we had an opportunity to discuss them later in this Symposium. I do find missing here a group of tumours originating from the intracerebral connective tissue. We have other brain tumours which up to the present we have regarded not as gliomatous but as malignant connective tissue tumours.

Dr. Zülch: This is a question we have discussed.

Dr. Ringertz: I only want to point out that among this group of vascular structures nothing has been said about the racemose angiomas. Is this because you want to refer to vascular tumours in general?

Dr. Zülch: Yes, and the sarcomas too, you see, Dr. Hamperl pointed out to me that only those tumours should be listed under the central nervous system and its structures, that were very characteristic of this organ. That means sarcomas, like the fibrosarcoma of the dura, which as we probably all agree occurs very similarly in other parts of the body, should not be listed here. They are included under the sarcomas, so perhaps we don't need them in this part of the classification. Is that correct?

Dr. Hamperl: Completely correct. We have here mesenchymal tumours, tumours of fibrous tissue and here a subgroup vascular tissue and haemangioma racemosum. If you see a slide without the surrounding tissue would you be able to say that it is a haemangioma racemosum? probably not, therefore it comes under vascular structures. The same applies to reticulosarcomas and fibrosarcomas and all the other types of sarcomas.

Dr. Zülch: Would you comment on the last group, Dr. Hamperl?

Dr. Hamperl: The last group is the paraganglia and we have only one tumour arising from paraganglia, either from the carotid body or the other paraganglia along the vascular parts to the typanum and it was proposed to make two subdivisions following the "Fascicle", the adenomatoid and angiomatoid.

Dr. Zülch: I miss the horrible name of chemodectoma.

Dr. Rubinstein: I was just going to propose it, Dr. Zülch, because I want to raise the question as to what is a paraganglioma. Many people include the paraganglioma under chromaffin tumours, in other words the pheochromocytomas, and there is a great deal of confusion. That is why the term chemodectoma which is confined to the carotid body tumours and glomus jugulare tumours is a useful one since it separates them very sharply from the chromaffin-producing tumours arising from the adrenals or from the organs of Zuckerkandl.

Dr. Zülch: Dr. Rubinstein, I think chemodectoma is not generally accepted yet, or at least it is confined to the United States. Etymologically it is a bad term because the tumours in pathology are usually named after tissues or cells. In my view we ought not to base our terminology on *site* like infundibuloma or function like chemodectoma, but if possible on tissues or cells.

Dr. Hamperl: May I ask, Dr. Rubinstein, if the name chemodectoma is really accepted, really widely used. This is a point, which is of importance.

Dr. Rubinstein: I really can't answer that question, Dr. Hamperl, as to how widely people use this particular term. The point about the carotid body tumours is that they have nothing to do with the chromaffin-producing cells, because chromaffin-producing cells are supposed to arise from neuroblasts, whereas the carotid body cells, the chemoreceptors, arise from mesodermal cells. The carotid body arises from the third pharyngeal arch. There is no relationship between the chromaffin-producing cells and these.

Dr. Hamperl: I think Willis has made a really good study of these tumours in one of the last issues of Cancer or another journal. I hate the word chemodectoma of course, and I completely agree with Dr. Zülch that it is not a good word. On the other hand I agree that if chemodectoma is widely used and there are people in the United States who know what chemodectoma is and use this name, we should put the name in just as we put in gemistocytic astrocytoma.

Dr. Zülch: Yes, but then we need more urgently glomus tumour in the same group. Even in the Cancer Seminar in Colorado Springs U. S. A.* the first name was "glomus tumour" with "chemodectoma" in brackets. And there were about 300 American pathologists. So from this I deduce that glomus tumour is better understood by American pathologists than chemodectoma.

Dr. Hamperl: There are very serious objections against the use of the word glomus tumour. Firstly we already have in our nomenclature the word glomus tumour in regard to glomus tumours of the skin. We can't have the same term in two places meaning two different tumours. Probably the use of the term glomus tumour for tumours of the skin is wider than the use of the name glomus tumour for carotid body tumours for which we have other good names. So I would be in favour putting in, reluctantly of course, chemodectoma, but leaving out glomus tumour.

Dr. Zülch: Yes, perhaps a note could be made, however, that in Germany for instance the neurosurgeons all know what a glomus tumour is. The pathologists all use the term glomus tumour. They don't talk about carotid body tumours, so at least let us have a little footnote, that this tumour corresponds to the glomus tumour of the clinician or something like that, otherwise the clinician will never understand what you mean by chemodectoma.

Dr. Hamperl: Could we not put in glomus caroticum tumour? Would this suit?

Dr. Zülch: Yes, alright. But the word glomus has to appear.

Dr. Hamperl: Glomus caroticum tumour.

Dr. Zülch: Carotid body and in bracket "glomus caroticum" tumour.

Unidentified: We have not however considered the jugulare tumours.

Dr. Zülch: Yes, they form a single entity.

Dr. Hamperl: Good, I will take both of them.

Dr. Zülch: ... Dr. Hamperl, in conclusion I as the chairman of this Symposium thank you for your very valuable contribution to our discussion. I think we all had the impression that this was a very fruitful session and that the collaboration was very cordial. We spoke very open and frankly and I think this is the best way to proceed. We know each other very well because of our contributions to the subject of brain tumours and therefore we can discuss and change our opinions very freely. Next we will have a discussion on the heredity of tumours in man by Dr. Koch.

---

* See: Cancer Seminar, Vol. II, Nr. 2 (1956).

b) The Contribution of Different Techniques to Classification

1. Genetics

The Genetics of Cerebral Tumours

By

G. Koch*

Amongst human brain tumours the inheritance of neurofibromatosis and tuberous sclerosis has been known for many years. Both diseases are classed as phakomatoses or hamartoblastoses because of the presence of the skin and eye changes which frequently accompany them.

A table may give a survey of the various clinical pictures which are grouped together under the heading "phakomatoses". I would like to say that this classification is taken from the chapter on "phakomatoses" which I have prepared for a hand-book of human genetics. Before I turn to the familial gliomatosis-glioblastomatosis as cerebral tumours in the narrow sense, I would like to bring to your notice a few findings in neurofibromatosis, tuberous sclerosis. *von Hippel-Lindau's* and *Sturge-Weber's* diseases which are important from the point of view of genetics. *Sturge-Weber's* syndrome has recently become the focus of attention of genetic interests in so far as in occasional cases chromosome abnormalities have been found in tissue cultures.

Neurofibromatosis is characterised by a very varied clinical picture. Its frequency according to different estimations varies between 1 : 2000 and 1 : 3000 in the average population. The inheritance is dominant or irregularly dominant. Both sexes are almost equally affected. The familial findings show a great intrafamilial variability. It stems from a developmental lability of the *anlage*.

In this regard neighbouring genes and also paratypical factors appear to be of significance. It is of interest that there are occasional families in which there is a certain similarity of tumour structure within the family.

The fertility of patients with neurofibromatosis is markedly diminished; according to recent American investigations about 52.7% (in men 41.3%, in woman 74.8%). The basis of this appears to be

---

* See: *Koch, G.*, Erbliche Hirngeschwülste. Zschr. menschl. Vererb. 29 (1949), 400—423. — *Koch, G.*, Beitrag zur Erblichkeit der Hirngeschw. Acta Gen. med. gem. III (1954), 170—191.

the more than average frequency of celibacy in the patients. This has important implications for genetics: if half of the trait carriers in one generation are eliminated so must the constancy of the incidence of the illness in the population be kept up through fresh mutation. The mutation rate is estimated at 1×10^{-4}, i. e. 100 mutating genes per million gametes. It is so far the highest mutation rate which has been estimated for an autosomal dominant characteristic. The *unilateral or bilateral acoustic neurinomas* are worthy of discussion. They are more frequent in women than in men. Bilateral acoustic neurinomas without neurofibromatosis are rare.

Unilateral acoustic neurinomas with neurofibromatosis are also infrequent. Both however are possible. The inheritance of bilateral acoustic neurinomas bound to neurofibromatosis has frequently been reported. Individual families allow recognition here also of an intrafamilial similarity.

The unilateral acoustic neurinoma occurs almost always sporadically. *Hauge-Harvald* (1960) found secondary cases in close relationship to the 106 probands only in three families thus in the remaining 103 families the acoustic neurinoma occured in isolation. The number of affected relatives amounted to 1090. This finding suggests that the unilateral acoustic neurinoma belongs to a special inherited type with weak penetrance.

Tuberous sclerosis is actually rarer than neurofibromatosis. Its frequency in the average population is estimated between 1 : 30,000 to 1 : 150,000. *Both sexes* are equally affected. The type of inheritance is dominant or irregularly dominant. In individual families a recessive inheritance cannot be excluded with certainty. The familial findings show in general a great intrafamilial variability; in individual families there is also a certain intra-familial similarity. The great phenotypical variability of tuberous sclerosis rests according to *Penrose* and others on the activity of a polyphenic head gene and the modified activity of the neighbouring gene.

The fertility of the trait carriers of tuberous sclerosis is reduced, according to a Danish investigation by *Borberg*, to 51%. In one generation therefore half of all *anlages* for tuberous sclerosis would be eliminated. The principal reason for this is the fact that in severe cases with epilepsy occuring in earliest childhood and with severe mental deficiency there is early confinement to an asylum. The mutation rate in England was estimated at $4—8 \times 10^{-6}$ i. e. 4—8 mutating genes per million gametes.

Von Hippel-Lindau's disease is inherited as dominant or irregularly dominant. Amongst these cases, 20% of the patients with angioblastoma of the cerebellum show angiomatosis of the retina,

26.9% of the pancreas and in 34.8% there are renal malformations (mostly cystic pancreas and cystic kidneys). *As well as these familial cases* the angioma of the cerebellum — like the unilateral acoustic neuroma in neurofibromatosis — in the majority of cases occurs sporadically. According to a collective study of *Krayenbühl* 6% of cases were familial. There is a very feeble tendency in the sporadic cases to simultaneous occurrence of angiomatosis of the retina and other visceral malformations. *In contrast to* the unilateral acoustic tumour the isolated occurence of angioblastoma of the cerebellum is a definite inherited disease entity.

Sturge-Weber's disease occurs predominately sporadically. In this regard we know of occasional familial findings, which suggest dominant or irregularly dominant or recessive inheritance. Aetiologically unsatisfactorily explained diseases with a predominantly sporadic occurence have in the last two years been investigated by chromosome studies where the chromosomes have been suspect as aetiological factors. So first *Hayward-Bower* (1960) reported that in a case of *Sturge-Weber's* disease a trisomia of the 22 acrocentral autosome was found. This finding was not confirmed in *Wilke's* investigation of 16 cases. Recently *Patau* and collaborator found in one case a chromosomal translocation (T). This finding showed that in *Sturge-Weber's* disease different aetiological factors were concerned. It could be mentioned that in neurofibromatosis and tuberous sclerosis also, complete investigations have been carried out. Their results were, however, as expected, negative. For brain and spinal cord tumours in general *Zülch* (1956) estimated for the same age group in the German population a fatality rate of 1 : 20 or 1 : 25,000. Out of this large group of cerebral tumours occuring sporadically in the family and doubtlessly not inherited, a group of familial cases has been for a long time recognized, which histologically belong predominantely to the gliomatosis-glioblastomatosis group. They have been observed in siblings or in two generations following upon one another.

In a family studied by me in 1943 the mother died of a glioma of the left parieto-occipital lobe. In the daughter there was a glioblastoma multiforme of the left parieto-temporal lobe and in the son a cystic glioblastoma of the right temporal lobe. In a more recent observation, three sisters died at the age of 50—54 years of glioblastoma multiforme, which in two of the sisters was confirmed histologically.

Topographically there is in these familial cases an infiltrating juxta-ventricular tumour localised in the depths of the brain. The sites of predilection were on the one hand the frontal — corpus callosal — temporal region and on the other the parieto-occipital region. The clinical picture is characterised by an acute onset and usually a course leading to death in a short time. The Danes, *Harvald-Hauge* who reject the possibility of inherited factors underlying this familial gliomatosis-glioblastomatosis group, consider the occurence of several cases in one family as coincidence. They support their conclusion by familial studies in which they found amongst 1813 relatives of 179 probands with glioblastoma only 5 secondary cases of intracranial tumour. In a control series of 249 probands without cerebral tumour there were on the other hand amongst 2288 relatives 10 secondary cases demonstrated. The death rate of 1.2% was not significantly different from the death rate of 0.8% in the control group. The findings of the Dutch investigator *van der Weil* conflicted with the Danish results. He found the death rate from glioma amongst the relatives of the tumour group 4 times higher than would have been expected. His material provided 100 glioma patients with 5262 relatives studied. 100 families with 2228 relatives served as a controlled series. This investigation established, apart from the observations to date, that the majority of familial cases are malignant gliomas, for which an inherited basis can be assumed.

The origin of the differing results lies in my opinion in the material, which *Hauge-Harvald* derived from the neurosurgical clinic in Copenhagen but in *van der Wiels's** cases was obtained from the University Neurological Clinic in Utrecht. *Zülch* has always insisted that malignant glioblastomas are to be found less frequently in neurosurgical clinics than, for example, in general pathological institutes and neurological clinics. So I would like on the basis of my own investigations to reject *van der Wiel's* postulation that familial gliomatosis-glioblastomatosis is a rare specific inherited type. As regards the initial phase of this familial gliomatosis-glioblastomatosis there is nothing yet completely clear. The predilection depends in all probability on a dysontogenetic factor. The assumption that an embryo with a defective enzyme exists dysontogenetically in the "initial phase" directs attention to the second stimulating factor which initiates the promotion phase. Because glioblastomas occur at the time of the hormonal changes of age and sex involution, as for example in the three sisters mentioned, one might imagine that hormonal factors initiate growth in the topographically predisposed areas.

* *Van der Wiel. H. J.*, Inheritance of Glioma. Elsevier Publ. Comp., Amsterdam-London-New York, 1960.

Discussion

Dr. Zülch: Thank you, Dr. Koch. The paper is open for discussion. — Would you like to say a few words on brain tumours in twins, because there are some concordant and some discordant examples in the literature? Are there any other questions or comments or suggestions to Dr. Koch?

Dr. Woolf: I would like to ask one thing, whether the occurance of a particular tumour in two siblings is significant or does it have to be in three before it becomes of interest; we have had one case of medulloblastoma occuring in two brothers and there is a case from Antwerp of two meningiomas of the foramen magnum in brothers. These were not mentioned. I wonder if that is because you have to have more than three before it is of statistical interest.

Dr. Zülch: I think there are quite a good many families where you have two members, two brothers or two sisters or two members of the same generation with brain tumours and Dr. Koch could not probably mention all of these. Dr. Koch would you care to comment on the question about the statistical significance, whether you need two or three.

Dr. Koch: It makes no difference. Two is enough in order to be statistically significant.

Dr. Woolf: The practical question is whether it is desirable to report for example two gliomas in siblings.

Dr. Koch: Yes, because brain tumours in twins are rather rare and familial occurances have been unfrequently observed, up to the present it is worth reporting every case observed.

Dr. Zülch: Would you like to comment on the twins?

Dr. Koch: The total number of reports of observations in twins are shown here. They show concordant occurance of medulloblastoma twice in uniovular twins and also gliomas in uniovular twins have been reported twice. Neuroblastoma of the retina has been reported once in uniovular twins. It is interesting that only cases in uniovular twins are reported.

Dr. Rubinstein: One of the twins that you mentioned here had a meningioma and the other a glioblastoma. What significance would you attach to this?

Dr. Koch: Yes, one has in individual cases assumed that a specific trait is inherited, for example in familial cases of gliomatosis or glioblastomatosis which is histologically similar. In other cases one presumes that a susceptability to brain tumours in general is inherited. This explains how uniovular twins with different types of brain tumour occur. But we must all bear in mind that the diagnosis may not have been made by the same pathologist in both of the twins.

Dr. Rubinstein: Yes, thank you.

Dr. Koch: I would like to conclude from my table that inheritance generally does not play a role in cerebral tumours and that there are only a few familial cases in which inheritance can be assumed — these are the familial gliomatosis and glioblastomatosis which I have referred to above. We are not in a position so far to produce a sufficiently large series of twins concerning a particular type of brain tumour. We have only a few binovular discordant twins in the glioma series. It is also possible to demonstrate in the gliomas, as has Van der Wiel from Holland, that the statistical correlation frequency of twinning and glioblastoma amounts to 1 in 35,000, i. e. amongst 35,000 glioblastomas there will be only one uniovular pair of twins.

Dr. Rubinstein: From this table Dr. Koch it is apparent that generally speaking there is no familial incidence in gliomas, generally apart from a small restricted group with definite evidence of a familial disposition. As regards the second table there is from the cases reported so far no definite indication that any one particular tumour has a special tendency to show a familial incidence.

Dr. Zülch: Thank you Dr. Rubinstein and Dr. Koch. Any other comments? I think, Dr. Koch has given us a very good bird's eye view of this extensive subject and one which we must take into account when we speak about the genesis of tumours. He has convinced us once more that all these questions of general cancerology can only be studied on an international basis, that means, that we need institutes where these family histories and case reports can be collected and it would be reasonable to ask the World Federation of Neurology also to support some work on this.

Thank you Dr. Koch. Now, next Dr. Luginbühl will speak on his observations on spontaneous brain tumours in animals.

2. Cerebral Tumours in Animals

A Comparative Study of Neoplasms of the Central Nervous System in Animals* **

By

H. Luginbühl

With 7 Figures

In the last 70 years there have been over 200 papers published on tumours of the C. N. S. in domestic animals, and most authors stress the rarity of such tumours. However, on the basis of our own experience and that reported in recent publications (*Frauchiger* and *Fankhauser,* 1957; *Dahme* and *Schiefer,* 1960; *McGrath,* 1960; *Smit,* 1961), we have formed the opinion that these tumours occur in the dog with a frequency and variety similar to that in man. The entire literature in this field fails to give a complete picture of the frequency, morphology and characteristics of C. N. S. tumours of animals. This can be explained by the paucity of any large series of cases (most articles being single case reports), the difficulty of interpretation of the histology of many tumours, and the absence of standardized nomenclature.

A statistical evaluation of the literature is therefore of little assistance. It is the task of the comparative neuropathologist to establish a broad biological basis for the understanding of C. N. S. tumours in all species including man. The classification and natural history of such tumours in man has been established by the well known work of *Bailey, Cushing, Hortega, Zülch, Kernohan* and others, based on a large number of cases. In order to obtain a sufficiently large series in animals, many colleagues in the commission of comparative Neuropathology (WFN) have contributed specimens to this study. We have 80 cases from our own material, and in addition over 250 C. N. S. tumours have been submitted by our colleagues for our opinion.

* This study was supported by Grant B 1916 of the National Institute for Nervous Diseases and Blindness, Bethesda 14, Maryland, USA and Swiss Nat. Foundation for Scientific Research.

** This paper is dedicated to Prof. Dr. *K. J. Zülch,* Director of the Max-Planck-Institute for Brain Research, Cologne-Merheim for his continuous help and encouragement.

The total series of 330 cases has been studied by standardized methods and each type of tumour has been compared with the corresponding tumour in man. Attempts have been made to evaluate tumour behaviour, localisation and architecture, the mesenchymal reactions within the tumour itself and the changes in the surrounding tissue. These aspects must be considered in relation to species, breed, age, sex and clinical symptomatology in order to view the tumours as a biological entity.

Table 1

Species	Neuro-ecto-dermal Tumours	Meso-dermal Tumours	Ecto-dermal Tumours	Teratoma	Metastases	Total
Cattle	8	21	1		2	33
Horse	2	6	5		1	14
Dog	69	49	28		37	183
Cat	4	40			8	52
Pig	3	7				10
Sheep		5				5
Goat	1					1
Mouse	2					2
Rat	2	3	7			12
Rabbit-Hare		1		1		2
Golden-Hamster	1					1
Elephant		1				1
Fowl	8	1				9
Budgerigar			5			5
Total	100	134	47	1	48	330

As methods of clinical investigation are more limited in dealing with animals than with man, it is obvious that pathological investigations must play a correspondingly greater part in any study.

The following survey of 330 tumours is based upon the classification proposed by *Zülch* (1956 a, 1956 b). Conclusions about the norm of a particular tumour were made not only on the characteristics of its constituent cells but also on the secondary changes seen within and surrounding the tumour. If these secondary changes were neglected, a large proportion of C. N. S. tumours could not be classified.

An analysis of the types of tumours and animal species affected is shown in the tables.

It has been possible to subclassify some 85% of all neuroectodermal tumours, but it must be admitted that there was doubt in some cases to which of two categories a particular tumour belonged because it contained some characteristics of each group.

The sex was known of 160 of 183 affected dogs, 85 being male and 75 female. Out of 163 dogs in which the breed was known, 57 were of brachycephalic breeds. This proportion is much greater than would be expected from the distribution of breeds which provide the general pathological material of any animal clinic. If only neuroectodermal tumours only are considered, the dominance among

Table 2. *Neuroectodermal Tumours*

Species	Medullo-blastoma	Spongio-blastoma	Oligodendro-glioma	Astrocytoma	Glioblastoma	Avian glioma	Unclass. Glioma	Ependymoma	Choroid plexus papilloma	Neurinoma	Gangliocytoma	Total
Cattle	1		1		3		2	1				8
Horse							1		1			2
Dog	5	3	33	4	5		7	3	7	1	1	69
Cat	1			1			1				1	4
Pig	1				1		1					3
Goat		1										1
Mouse			1		1							2
Rat							2					2
Golden Hamster							1					1
Fowl						8						8
Total	8	4	35	5	10	8	15	4	8	1	2	100

brachycephalic breeds becomes more striking as 40 out of 62 belonged to this group (30 Boxers, 10 Bulldogs, Boston Terriers and Bull Terriers).

We did not find any predisposition to C. N. S. tumours in other breeds of dogs.

Of 159 affected dogs in which the age was known, 19 (13%) were young dogs (1—4 years), 61 (38%) were mature adult dogs between 5 and 8 years and 79 (49%) were old dogs beween 9 and 15 years.

The Neuroectodermal Tumours (Table 2)

The 8 neoplasms classified under the general heading of *medulloblastoma* resemble human medulloblastomas in the majority of the morphological characteristics. 6 were situated in the cerebellum and 2 in the autonomic nervous system. The age of the animals affected corresponds to that of human patients with the same disorder. 6 were young animals, one was a young adult dog and the age of one was unknown.

Similarity to human *spongioblastomas* was seen in 4 neoplasms, 2 of which were in the cerebellum (dog) and one in the optic nerve (goat). In one case, accurate localisation could not be made on the material provided. No further comment can be made about this group at present.

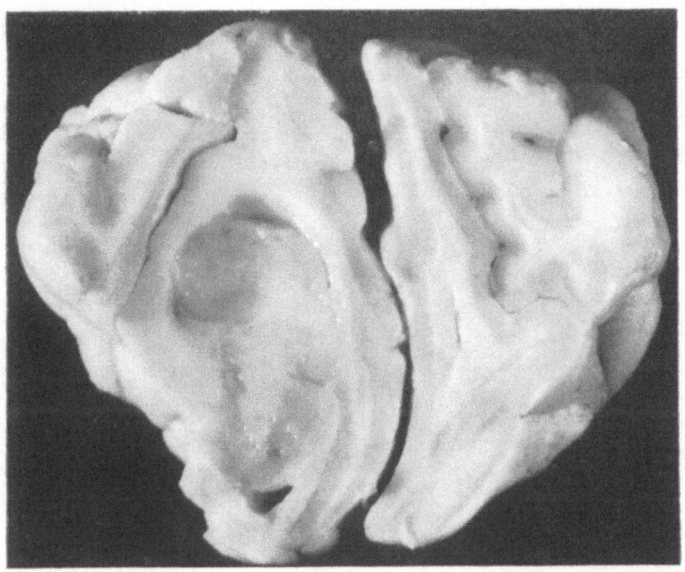

Fig. 1. Oligodendroglioma right frontal lobe (4524). Boxer, 9 years old, male.

In 35 cases (35% of all neuroectodermal tumours) the tumour proved to be an *oligodendroglioma*: 33 of these were in dogs, and one each in cow and mouse (*Cottier* and *Luginbühl*, 1961). The brachycephalic breeds of dogs provided 27 cases or 82% (23 Boxers, 2 Boston Terriers, 2 Bulldogs). Other breeds were represented by single cases only. Even considering the wide spread of the source of the material, it appears likely that some brachycephalic breeds have a predisposition to this type of tumour. With 3 exeptions, the age of onset of symptoms was between 5 and 11 years i. e. in the middle and old groups. The tumour could be localised in 32 cases: frontal and olfactory lobes, 12; base of brain and brain-stem, 8; temporal lobes including piriform area, 8; occipital and parietal lobes, 4. In many instances the oligodendrogliomas arise in the white matter and grow outwards toward the surface of the brain. In 18 cases the tumour was adjacent to a ventricle or even growing through its ependyma. In 12 cases the tumour infiltrated the leptomeninges. In oligodendrogliomas of dogs, there is extensive proliferation of capillary endothelium which gives a glomerular appearance. This mesodermal reaction appears often at the junction of tumour tissue with normal brain and with areas of cystic degeneration. Calcification has not been seen. In many of the cases metastases are distributed along the c. s. f. pathways.

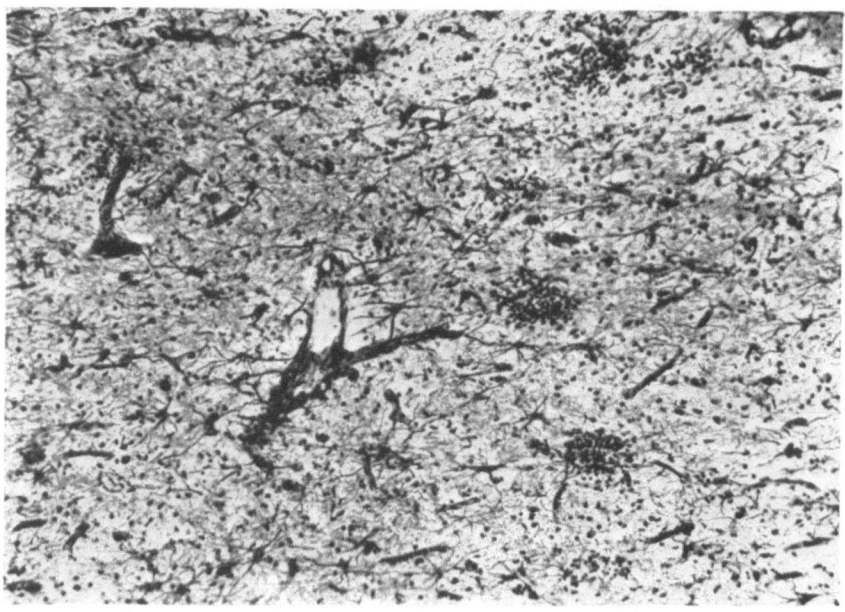

Fig. 2. Astrocytoma piriform area (4055). Bulldog, 9 year old, male. Fibrillary astrocytes, sucker feet, recent hemorrhages. Maurer impregnation, 120 ×.

Astrocytomas comprised only 5 cases of this series, and therefore appear to be relatively uncommon. 4 were seen in dogs (3 in brachy-cephalic breeds) and 1 in a cat.

No tumour comparable to the human astroblastoma was found.

10 cases of this series were *glioblastomas* (5 in dogs, 3 in cattle, 1 in a pig, and 1 in a mouse). This diagnosis is based upon the in-filtrative-destructive growth, pleomorphic cellularity, degenerative changes, abnormal blood vessels and haemorrhages.

A degree of pleomorphism similar to that of the human glio-blastoma multiforme was not observed.

In table 2, the heading "unclassified gliomas" implies that further subclassification of these tumours cannot be made with present knowledge.

2 neoplasms situated adjacent to a ventricle had a similar appearance to the nodules of tuberose sclerosis in man.

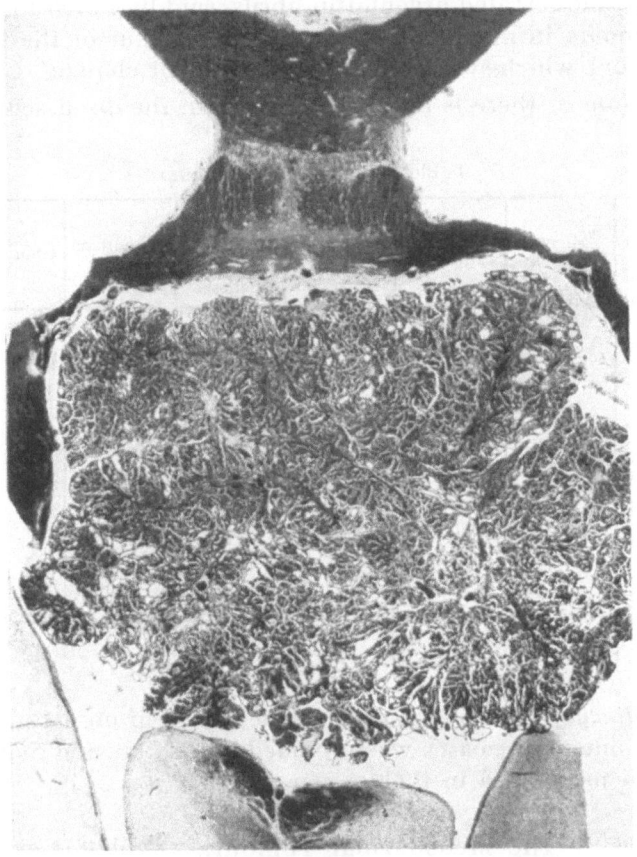

Fig. 3. Papilloma of choroid plexus of III. ventricle producing hydrocephalus (4289). White Cairn Terrier Dog, 2 years old. Luxol fast blue cresylviolet. Low power magnification. Case submitted by *J. B. M. Gellatly*, Edinburgh.

In fowls, a *multiple gliomatous process* may occur sporadically, and has been fully described in the classical work of *Jackson* (1954).

As only 4 *ependymomas* are listed in table 2, it should be mentioned that a few of the tumours classified as oligodendrogliomas and glioblastomas show some of the characteristics of ependymomas.

The 8 tumors of the choroid plexus have the following localisation: 2 in the lateral ventricles, 3 in the 3rd ventricle, and 3 in the 4th ventricle. The 7 dogs (including 4 Terriers) with *plexus papillomas* cover all age groups.

Neurinomas: 18 cases of neoplasms of cranial and peripheral nerves were found in this series, but it is our opinion that they are of mesodermal origin and might be called perineural fibroblastomas. However, the serrated argentaffin fibrils, said by *Zülch* to be typical of neurinoma in man, were found in one tumour of the trigeminal nerve (dog) which was undergoing malignant change.

Pinealomas: there is no pineal tumour in the discussed series.

Table 3. *Mesodermal Tumours*

Species	Menin-gioma	Vascular tumours	Perineural fibro-blastoma	Sarcoma and reticulo-endo-thelioses	Chondroma Lipoma	Chordoma	Total
Cattle	1		7	13			21
Horse		1		5			6
Dog	16	4	9	19		1	49
Cat	32	2	1	5			40
Pig		1		4	2		7
Sheep	1			4			5
Rat				3			3
Hare				1			1
Elephant			1				1
Fowl			1				1
Total	50	8	19	54	2	1	134

Gangliocytomas have very infrequently been observed. The material of one of our cases was provided by *Dahme* and *Schiefer,* and has been mentioned in their paper (1960).

The Mesodermal Tumours (Table 3)

Meningiomas: of all intracranial and intraspinal tumours in animals, meningiomas have been described most frequently and most accurately. Out of 50 cases of meningiomas, the majority were in cats (32 cases). Although some cases occured in younger age groups, most of them were in old animals.

Fig. 4. Gangliocytoma, cerebellum left of midline (3996). Shepherd, 4 years old, male, Trichome *(Goldner)*, 430 ×, Case submitted by Drs. *E. Dahme* and *B. Schiefer,* Munich.

Fig. 5. Multiple meningiomas (4092). Cat, 5 years old, male. Left: Dura inside. Meningiomas along falx cerebri and tentorium cerebelli. Right: Meningiomas seen along base of brain, pineal area and between the hemispheres.

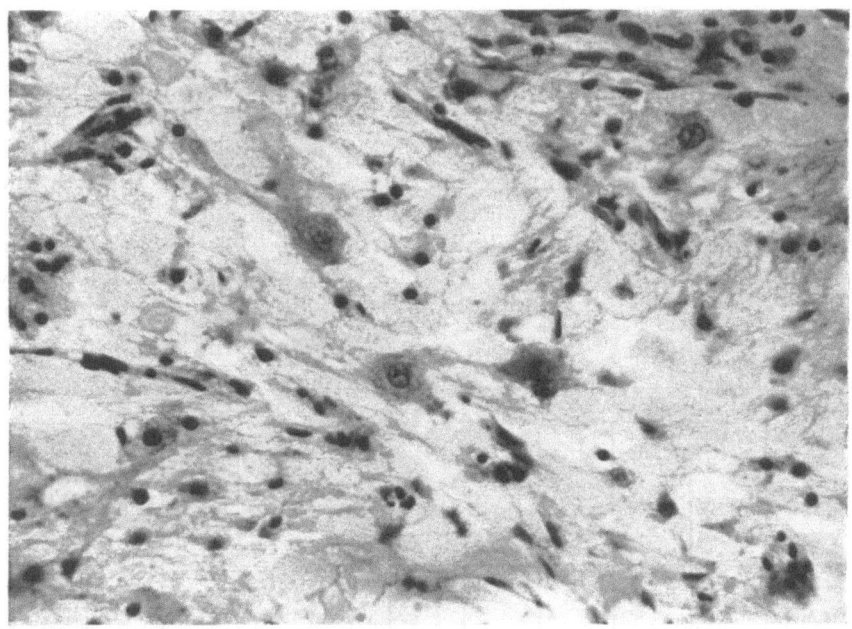

Fig. 4.

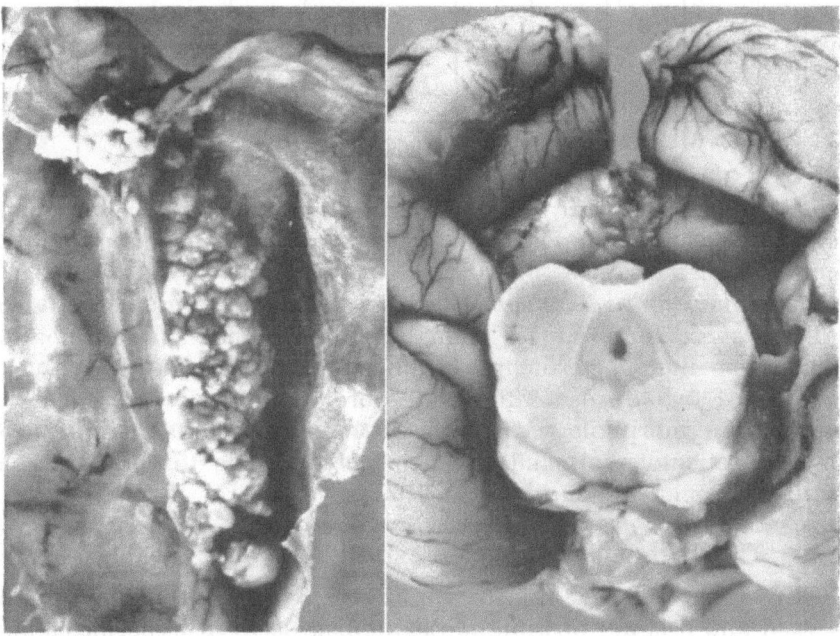

Fig. 5.

In striking contrast to the localisation of meningiomas in man, was a predilection for the tela choroidea of the third ventricle, the tumours running from the pineal area along the vena magna cerebri to the anterior end of the 3rd ventricle (*Luginbühl*, 1961). This localisation was observed in 18 cases. One third of these 18 cases showed additional meningiomas in other sites. With the exception of the angiomatous variety, all types seen in man were found.

Malformations and neoplasms of the blood vessels were seen in 8 cases (horse, dog, cat and pig). They consisted of morphologically inactive telangiectatic hamartomas, a cavernoma and haemangio-

Table 4

Species	Ectodermal Tumours				Metastases							
	Chromophobe pituitary adenoma	Chromophile pituitary adenoma	Unclass. ectodermal tumours	Total	Teratoma	Carcinoma different origin	Carcinoma mammary gland	Carcinoma ethmoid area	Sarcoma different origin	Melanoma	Total
Cattle		1	1	2		2					2
Horse	4	1		5		1					1
Dog	24	4		28		10	13	9	2	3	37
Cat						1	3	2	1	1	8
Rat	5	2		7							
Rabbit					1						
Budgerigar	3	2		5							
Total	36	10	1	47	1	14	16	11	3	4	48

endotheliomas. In two dogs hamartoid capillary and venous malformation in the hippocampus were found causing massive intracerebral haemorrhage.

Sarcomas and reticuloendothelioses: malignant mesodermal neoplasms were found in 54 animals of 8 different species (not including malignant perineural fibroblastomas).

Almost two thirds of the total were tumours of the reticulosis group. The morphology of many of these granulomatous and neoplastic reticuloendothelial lesions is comparable to the cases described in man by *Wilke* (1950, 1951) and others.

The Ectodermal and Metastatic Tumours (Table 4)

In old horses and rats the pituitary gland is often greatly enlarged and it is not possible to distinguish between hyperplasia and neoplasia with certainty. Most lesions classified as tumours show abnormal architecture and cell pleomorphism. Out of the 46 *pituitary adenomas,* 10 were chromophile.

Final Remarks

The organ of origin and species distribution of 48 *metastatic C. N. S. tumours* is shown in table 4.

1. The nature of the tumour-bearing tissue in animal and man may now be contrasted.

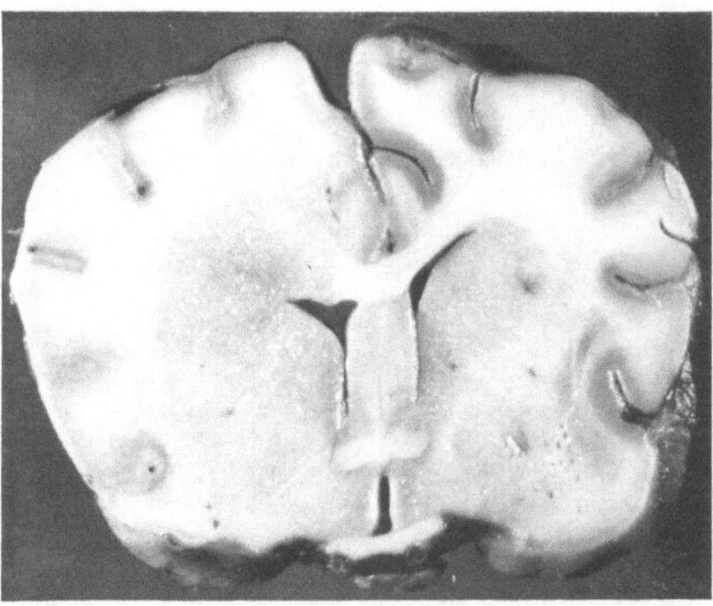

Fig. 6. Adventitial sarcoma (2058). Airedale Terrier, 14 years old, female. Large undefined tumour mass involving central white matter, corpus callosum and caudate nucleus of right hemisphere. Meningeal infiltration.

The present animal series is 330 cases, of which 30% are neuroectodermal, 41% are mesodermal, 14% ectodermal and 15% metastatic.

The analysis of 6000 human cases by *Zülch* (1960) provides the following figures: neuroectodermal 50.9%; mesodermal 23.2%; ectodermal 12.4%; metastatic 4.0%; miscellaneous space-occupying lesions 5.8%; unclassified blastomas 3.7%.

In *Zülch's* series, 14% of all neuroectodermal tumours are oligodendrogliomas, compared with 48% in the dog in our series.

In man, sarcomas comprise 2.7% of all intracranial tumours, whereas the corresponding figure in our animal series is 17.0%.

Evaluation of a larger number of animal cases may well alter the pattern of distribution apparent in this series.

2. It was not possible to classify 15% of neuroectodermal tumours in terms applied to human C. N. S. tumours, even though most important techniques were used and we had the advantage of consultation with Professor *Zülch*.

3. The relative frequency of occurence of gliomas, especially oligodendrogliomas, in some brachycephalic breeds of dogs is con-

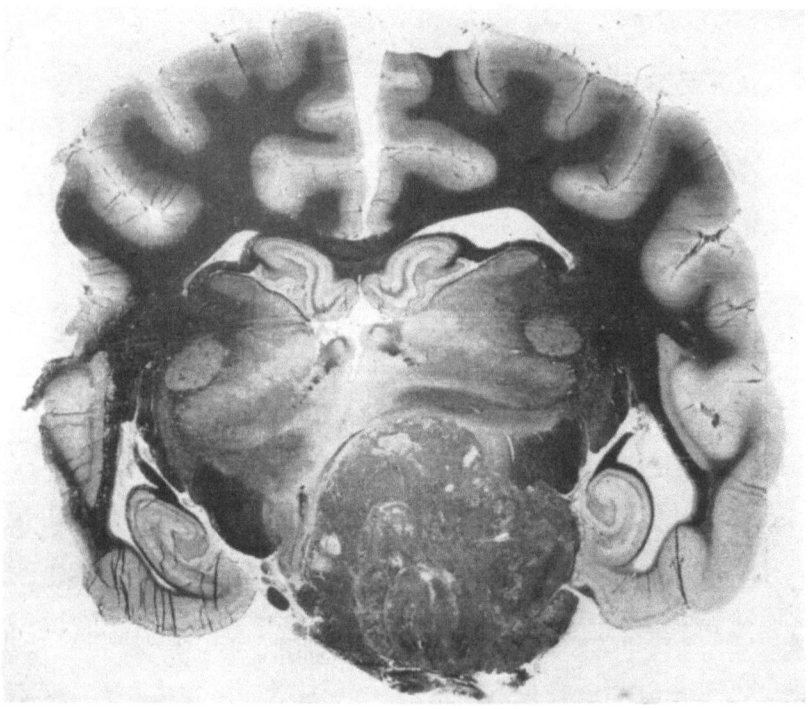

Fig. 7. Pituitary adenoma, chromophobe and foetal type (3077). Dachshund, 4 years old, male. Tumour growing into diencephalon and along base of brain.

firmed. The reason for this association will be discussed in later publications.

4. Some differences of morphology and localisation were presented. In many instances, in different types of tumours, small round cells were seen as perivascular infiltrates or occuring as foci independent of blood vessels. Such cells, which are morphologically compatible with lymphoid elements, were noted within the tumour substance, and in the surrounding tissue.

Acknowledgement

An extensive study of neoplasms of the central nervous system was made possible through the valuable contribution of cases from the colleagues named on the list.

Prof. *van den*		Dr. *Innes,*	New York
Akker,	Utrecht	Dr. *Jones,*	Boston
Prof. *Barboni,*	Perugia	Dr. *Jones,*	London
Dr. *Beach,*	London	Dr. *Jubb,*	Guelph
Dr. *Beattie,*	Edinburgh	Dr. *Kennedy,*	Davies (Cal.)
Prof. *Cohrs,*	Hanover	Dr. *Kersting,*	Bonn
Dr. *Cotchin,*	London	Prof. *Köhler,*	Wien
Dr. *Cottier,*	Bern	Dr. *Markson,*	Weybridge
Dr. *Dahme,*	München	Prof. *Oettel,*	Ludwigshafen
Dr. *Davies,*	Liverpool	Dr. *Osborne,*	Bristol
Dr. *Done,*	Weybridge	Prof. *Pallaske,*	Giessen
Dr. *Dunn,*	Bethesda	Dr. *Pilleri,*	Bern
Dr. *Gellatly,*	Edinburgh	Dr. *Sandersleben,*	Giessen
Dr. *Guazzi,*	Anvers	Dr. *Saunders,*	Philadelphia
Dr. *Harding,*	Weybridge	Dr. *Schiefer,*	München
Dr. *Hartley,*	Wellington	Prof. *Sedlmeyer,*	München
Prof. *Hauser,*	Bern	Prof. *Stünzi,*	Zürich
Dr. *Head,*	Edinburgh	Prof. *Zülch,*	Köln
Dr. *Howell,*	Liverpool		

The author and Prof. Dr. *E. Frauchiger,* Secretary of the Commission for Comparative Neuropathology wish to thank the contributors for their valuable help.

References

Cottier, H., and *H. Luginbühl,* Oligodendrogliom des Großhirns bei einer weißen Maus. Acta neuropath. *1* (1961), 198—200. — *Dahme, E.,* and *B. Schiefer,* Intracranielle Geschwülste bei Tieren. Zbl. Vet. med. 7 (1960), 341—363. — *Frauchiger, E.,* and *R. Fankhauser,* Vergleichende Neuropathologie des Menschen und der Tiere. Springer-Verlag, Berlin, 1957. — *McGrath, J. T.,* Neurologic Examination of the Dog. Sec. Ed. Lea & Febiger, Philadelphia, 1960. — *Jackson, C.,* Studies in comparative Neuropathology. I. Gliomas of the domestic fowl: their pathology with special reference to histogenesis and pathogenesis, and their relationship to other diseases. Onderstepoort. J. vet Res. *26* (1954), 501—597. — *Luginbühl, H.,* Studies on Meningiomas in cats. Amer. J. vet. Res. 22 (1961), 1030—1040. — *Smit, J. D.,* The lesions found at autopsy in dogs and cats which manifest clinical signs referable to the central nervous system. J. S. Afr. Vet. Med. Ass. *32* (1961), 47—55. — *Wilke, G.,* Über primäre Reticuloendotheliosen des Gehirns, mit besonderer Berücksichtigung bisher unbekannter eigenartiger granulomatöser Hirnprozesse. Dtsch. Zschr. Nervenhk. *164* (1950), 332—380. — *Wilke, G.,* Über Retothelsarkome des Gehirns. Verh. Dtsch. Ges. Path. *35* (1951),

178—183. — *Zülch, K. J.,* Die Hirngeschwülste in biologischer und morphologischer Darstellung. 2. Aufl., J. A. Barth-Verlag, Leipzig, 1956 a. — *Zülch, K. J.,* Biologie und Pathologie der Hirngeschwülste in Olivecrona H. und W. Tönnis Handbuch der Neurochirurgie Bd. III, 1—702. Springer-Verlag, Berlin, 1956. — *Zülch, K. J.,* The present state of the classification of intracranial tumours and its value for the neurosurgeon. Rev. bras. cir. *40* (1960), 247—264 and in: The biology and treatment of intracranial tumors, Ch. Thomas, Springfield 1962.

Discussion

Dr. Zülch: I think we are full of admiration for what you have attained in these two or three years, I don't know how many there actually were and I don't know whether I should not admire more the enthusiasm with which you hunted out these rare tumours, finding a case here and there at meetings or in veterinary journals or the accuracy with which you have worked through your material. May I conclude by saying that we all look forward to see your material condensed in a book. Now, the paper is open to discussion, and I think many of you would like now to see all the various slides and discuss the various problems of tumours i. e. whether these oligodendrogliomas are truely oligodendrogliomas or not and whether they were all correctly classified.

He followed a certain line in his classification, similar to our own and you may assume that Dr. Luginbühl has usually followed our descriptions. We saw most of the cases together. We had to take something as a basis to begin with. May be that when Dr. Luginbühl gains his own experience in the course of the years he will classify them differently, but we both agreed that at the beginning we ought to make the animal tumour series comparable to our own. Thank you so much, Dr. Luginbühl. The paper is open to discussion.

Dr. Hamperl: I was also very impressed. One always has to speak in pictures. For example I know the plants in this country and when I go up to the Alps, there are the same plants, the same families, but looking a little different. And I have this feeling too in comparing tumours in animals with tumours of men, they are of the same sort, but there are differences. The second point I would like to make is, isn't your table also an artificial selection? For example, consider the frequency in the different species of animals such as the dog and pig. The dog lives out his life in a friendly family as man's best friend, whereas the pig is killed in childhood and very seldom lives up to his natural end. The same is true for the cat where you have very many tumours, so I ask you, isn't the frequency very much dependent on the age at which you kill your animals?

Dr. Zülch: I would like you to comment on this, because this has been a matter of discussion for a long time between us. Would you kindly, Dr. Luginbühl?

Dr. Luginbühl: I fully agree with you. This an artificial selection in so far as all domestic animals do not reach their physiological senility so we only get tumours of their childhood. We can only study the pathology of infancy. But in dogs and cats it is different, and I think that I said that tumours of the central nervous system in dogs occur with the same frequency and variability as they do in man. Naturally, many things are again very different. We do not have the same possibilities for clinical investigation and examination as you have. Naturally in many areas or for many people the dog is the best friend and they are prepared to pay bills to the veterinary surgeon but in many cases they are not and very often when the first symptoms are noticed the animal is put to sleep by euthanasia and in some institutes where people are interested in brain pathology, many brains are removed and then one finds a lot of tumours and other lesions in routine autopsies, whereas in other institutes they just don't care and usually throw the material away, so this again adds to the artificial selection of the material, but I think there is no way out of this situation. An important reason for continuing the study is that for the last 30 years a tremendous effort has been made to study experimental tumours, but only very little to study spontaneous pathology or spontaneous diseases in animals which are not financially rewarding. Therefore I think, it is high time to start comparative pathology, not only neuropathology, but in all other fields, cardiovascular etc. We should study all these important dieseases occuring spontaneously in animals, but we know already that practically all types of tumours seen in man can occur in animals.

Dr. Netsky: May I ask a question. There is a factor of selection here. Are these animals who have had symptoms of cerebral disease or are they routine autopsies?

Dr. Luginbühl: Both, I cannot give you the percentage of either. But more than half of them were put to sleep or died from nervous symptoms and were autopsied and another proportion, I think about 10 to 20% — this is not an exact figure — have been found on routine autopsy. It is very interesting that sometimes I have found rather large tumours in animals showing no symptoms what so ever.

Dr. Netsky: Another question. Those observations of the brachycephalic dog having a high incidence of brain tumours is certainly interesting and I wonder whether you know any work on human material in relation to size of cranium. I am just not familiar with it.

Dr. Luginbühl: No, I don't know any human work on that.

Dr. Zülch: Would you think that the brachycephalic races and particularly that the boxer dogs are degenerate?

Dr. Luginbühl: No, I think this is a bad word to use. I would not use the word degeneration. I cannot explain to you what brachycephalis is, but I think it is wrong to call it just degeneration. If you look at a boxer apart from the short nose it does not look at all degenerated.

Dr. Zülch: Thank you, Dr. Luginbühl. Dr. Rubinstein?

Dr. Rubinstein: There is one comment I would like to make on Dr. Luginbühl's remarkable series. One thing that struck me is the remarkable resemblance of these tumours to human equivalents, and I think this is extremely instructive. But I am impressed by the fact , that whereas the histology is so very similar, the incidence is in some ways so very dissimilar. The high incidence of oligodendrogliomas among dogs is quite in opposition to what we have in man. The high incidence of mesodermal tumours in the cat compared with the low incidence of gliomas is again very striking. And particularly the third ventricle meningiomas which are excessively rare in man. There are obviously some obscure factors involved here.

Dr. Luginbühl: May I make a remark about the third ventricle meningiomas in the cat. When I studied for one year in Boston, I reported a series of 550 animals, in whom I took out every brain routinely and tried to examine them as completely as possible. And in a series of 155 cats which I opened routinely I found 7 intraventricular meningiomas and none of them showed symptoms, though some of them were of a considerable size in comparison with the size of the brain. We had not a single case in Berne. I have not had a single case from any other European country except the region of Edinburgh, from which I have had another 8 cases. I cannot explain it, but it is just a fact. I know in Philadelphia a few cases have been reported also.

Dr. Rubinstein: May I just ask one more question regarding one of the pictures you projected. I refer to the tumour of a cat which was interpreted as a medulloblastoma. You showed these very remarkable rosettes. I don't know whether this is the time to discuss the diagnosis of these cases, but I wonder whether this could not possibly be a malignant ependymoma.

Dr. Luginbühl: I am sure one can raise this question. We discussed the case together, Dr. Zülch and myself.

Dr. Zülch: Yes.

Dr. Rubinstein: I saw these remarkable rosettes with tubules and cavities, and that seems to me unlikely to be an medulloblastoma.

Dr. Luginbühl: On the other hand you have seen the very high number of mitotic figures.

Dr. Rubinstein: Oh, yes, it is a malignant tumour, I agree, and I wonder if this could not be a malignant ependymoma.

Dr. Zülch: Well, there could be some discussion on this or that tumour. We will just take the general figures for granted now. Dr. Schiefer, you want to make some remarks.

Dr. Schiefer: I want to say that the metastases of brain tumours of dogs occur more often than your material suggests. We have collected many metastases in the last 2 years. Another point, we have two cases of oligodendrogliomas with calcification. I think it also occurs in dogs. And a question about the spongioblastoma from the goat which was demonstrated. I have stained it with Gomori's silver method and I saw in most parts a structure like a retothelial sarcoma.

Dr. Zülch: Yes, we will have to see that tonight in the slide session.

Dr. Schiefer: Finally another question. Were the perivascular lymphoid tumours only in the brain, or were there also generalised cases?

Dr. Luginbühl: Concerning the metastases I fully agree with you. Most contributors of material just send cases they think are neuroectodermal. But certainly metastases are rather frequent, and concerning a spongioblastoma, as Dr. Zülch said, we have done all these stains too and we have seen that too, but in most parts, also in the tumour in the eye, there are areas typical, I think, of spongioblastoma and oligodendroglioma.

Dr. Schiefer: The mesodermal...

Dr. Luginbühl: Oh yes, I did not want to make any remarks about them, because we will talk on Friday about sarcomas, but I have also cases with me.

Dr. Zülch: Dr. Calvo wanted to comment on this.

Dr. Calvo: I find this comparative pathology of brain tumours extremely interesting and I think that it will be really important to compare on the basis also of comparative histology. A very important fact that should be taken as a working hypothesis is why in dogs there are no or very few glioblastomas and many oligodendrogliomas. This is really striking. And a very interesting fact about the astrocytes of the dog is that they have the largest sucker feet of astrocytes of all the animals I know. This may be a sort of protection against degeneration of the glial cells producing tumours. That would be a very interesting point to study.

Dr. Zülch: Thank you very much, Dr. Calvo. I think this is a very good idea to follow and you may be sure that Dr. Luginbühl in the future will try to do his best in adopting all the methods available, but the snag was really that in collecting these tumours he often found them in old collections and only as H. E. sections or an old Van Gieson stain. It was very difficult for him to work on these, the blocks and fresh material not being available.

Dr. Calvo: May I suggest Dr. Luginbühl, that you should stain with this idea as many specimens as you can with sublimate gold chloride which gives you the best staining of the gliovascular structure.

Dr. Luginbühl: But should not the material be fresh? We just get formalin-fixed material and often it has been in formalin for months or years, and the results we have got so far have been very poor.

Dr. Calvo: I can offer you some help in this and give you some methods that would demonstrate the gliovascular relations in formalin material.

Dr. Luginbühl: Thank you very much.

Dr. Zülch: I think Dr. Liss whom I have not welcomed yet and who is just visiting our institute would also like to comment. Would you?

Dr. Liss: Thank you very much. I just would like to ask one question. I hope I am not jumping the gun. Would you care to comment shortly about the morphological correlations between the spontaneous tumours in dogs and those which occur after induction with methyl-cholanthrene, especially in relation to the so-called mixed tumours in dogs.

Dr. Zülch: Could we postpone the question until after Dr. Netsky has spoken. Perhaps that would be better. Are there any other comments or questions? I think that we can again thank you very much, Dr. Luginbühl.

3. Experimental Production of Brain Tumours

Experimental Induction and Transplantation of Brain Tumors in Animals

By

M. G. Netsky

With 2 Figures

Gliomas may be induced in some strains of mice by intracerebral implantation of small pellets of carcinogens such as methylcholanthrene or benzpyrene. A latent period of 4 months to 2 years may elapse before the tumors are clinically evident. This length of exposure of the brain is relatively long in the life span of the mouse (usually a little more than 2 years). Neoplasms occuring earlier than 4 months after implantation are often sarcomas. The presence of an experimentally induced glioma in the mouse is easily recognized by paralytic or ataxic motor signs. The brain tumor may then be harvested and grown in successive transplants in the subcutaneous tissue, brain, or eye of homologous animals. Transplants are generally less successful in heterologous animals, in tissue culture or in the allantoic membrane of the chick egg.

Various gliomas may be produced having a striking histologic resemblance to those occurring in man. Study of these experimental tumors and their subsequent transplants has resulted in certain conclusions which will be critically examined.

1. *Species and strain of animal are important factors in the induction of experimental brain tumors; genetic factors play a role in determining the incidence of gliomas.* Attempts to induce brain tumors in rats, rabbits, guinea pigs and dogs have been uniformly unsuccessful (*Zimmerman* and *Arnold,* 1943). The mouse is the species used for induction of gliomas, but different strains have various degrees of susceptibility. *Zimmerman* and *Arnold* (1944), for example, using identical methods, induced gliomas in 24% of C3H mice, 56% of ABC albinos, 48% of Bagg albinos, 29% of C 57 blacks, 18% of A albinos, and only 10% of the dba strain. Unfortunately, crossbreeding experiments did not yield definitive results, and it must be concluded that the responsible genetic factors are probably multiple.

2. *Individual resistance to induction of brain tumors occurs under identical conditions.* In a large series, brain tumors will seldom appear in more than 50% of animals. Factors responsible for this resistance must reside within the individual if the genetic constitution is carefully controlled. The same pellet taken from an unsuccessful implant may be used successfully in another animal; hence the failure is not inherent in the carcinogen. Unfortunately, little information is available concerning factors of individual resistance. The mechanisms of resistance may well be more important than study of the tumors themselves.

3. *The site of implantation is a partial determinant of the type of glioma induced; the cells exposed to the carcinogen are a factor in determining which neoplasm is produced.* A medulloblastoma may occur when the carcinogenic pellet is placed in the cerebellum. Ependymoma is likely to result if the pellet is inserted close to the ependymal lining. Glioblastoma multiforme, oligodendroglioma and astrocytoma occur most often with carcinogens in the white matter. Most often, however, the tumors are "mixed" in the sense of simultaneous presence of different cells or groups of cells — astrocytic. spongioblastic, ependymal, oligodendroglial or unidentifiable. This situation is readily understandable. The carcinogen diffuses outward, and many cells surrounding the pellet absorb the material. It would be highly unlikely that each cell would be of the same type. Even if this improbable event occured, evidence has not been presented that similar cells in the brain always give rise to tumors of the same nature. Does an astrocyte induced to neoplasia always give rise to an astrocytoma? An affirmative answer is taken as an article of faith, but proof is lacking.

Recent work of *Koenig* et coll. (1961) suggests that reparative oligodendroglia may become fibrillary astrocytes. It is indeed difficult in many cases to distinguish an astrocytic from an oligodendroglial cell, whether by light or electron microscopy. In addition, it is notable that exceptions are found to the statements first cited in this section. Pellets near the ependyma induce various gliomas, although ependymomas often occur. The possibility of all glial cells being multi-potential in the neoplastic process cannot be dismissed. This potential has little in common with the developing nervous system. The frequent assumption that neoplasia follows the cellular path used by the embryonic nervous system has little evidence for it, but is implicit in the concept, for example, that a spongioblast is a de-differentiated astrocyte. Even those persons who agree with *Ewing* (1940) that "oncology is not a department of embryology" tend to apply their knowledge of the developing nervous system to neoplasms.

4. *Local tissue resistance to growth of gliomas is low: failure of these tumors to grow extra-cerebrally is not dependent on the "soil".* A frequently used site for homologous transplantation is the subcutaneous tissue of the mouse. Gliomas in this location usually grow readily. The nature of the transplant has an effect on growth: tumors appear more rapidly from suspensions of cells than from solid pieces. Gliomas will also grow in other parts of the body (Table 1). If an intravenous suspension of glioma is injected in the tail vein of a homologous mouse, tumors may be found in lungs,

Table 1. *Location of metastases after intravenous injection of suspension of tumor cells*

Mouse	Location of metastases
1	Lungs, pelvis of kidney, extra-thoracic region, lymph node.
2	Fallopian tube and pelvic region.
3	None seen.
4	Lungs, diaphragm, adrenals, subcu- taneous tissue of snout, extra-thoracic region, cardiac chambers.
5	None seen.
6	Lungs.
7	None seen.
8	Lungs.
9	Lungs.
10	None seen.

kidney, adrenal glands, lymph-nodes, etc. (Fig. 1). Most organs of the body therefore allow growth of gliomas, as is true in human beings. The rarity of metastasis of gliomas then is inherent in the tumors rather than the tissue in which they grow.

The cause of the inability of gliomas to metastasize is their failure to penetrate blood vessels. Glial cells are never seen in the vascular system unless mechanically or experimentally inserted; the mechanism of their failure to penetrate vessels is unknown. In un- published experiments, the hyalouronidase content of mouse glio- mas was compared with sarcomas and mammary carcinomas, but a significant difference was not found. Hyalouronidase was mixed with suspensions of glial cells and inoculated subcutaneously but this technic failed to promote metastases. The assumption that glio- mas lack some chemical factor present in metastasizing tumors may still be valid.

5. *Despite low tissue resistance, the rate of growth of gliomas under controlled conditions is extremely variable; unknown growth factors exist in the tumor or in the host.* Report has been made (*Netsky* and coll., 1956) of the effects of radiation on the growth of induced gliomas. Growth was determined in these studies by measuring the size of the subcutaneous tumor in 3 dimensions. The transplant was a small piece of tumor from a previous transplant. Control studies of the rate of growth of unirradiated tumors revealed wide variability (Fig. 2); a tumor more than doubled in size in 2 days in one animal, barely enlarged in another for 11 days and then rapidly increased in volume, and in a third animal, the

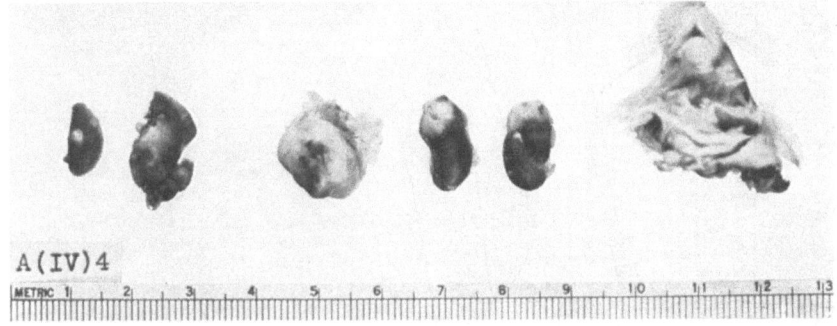

Fig. 1. Some of the sites of localization of tumor are seen in various organs of a mouse injected intravenously with a suspension of glial cells. The tissues from left to right are: right lung, left lung, ribs with overlying mass, right kidney and adrenal, left kidney and adrenal, undersurface of head (note asymmetric snout caused by bulging tumor) Each of these structures contains metastatic nodules.

tumor failed to grow. Variable growth in these experiments might have been related to heterogeneity of small transplants; some portions possibly were necrotic, whereas others might contain large numbers of viable cells.

To overcome this objection, the following previously unpublished experiments were performed in the C3H and A albino strains of mice, using an undifferentiated glioma and an ependymoma. Approximately 1 gm. of tumor tissue was placed in a test tube with 5 ml. of isotonic saline solution. The contents of the tube were then homogenized for 30 seconds with a rotating plunger revolving at 300 rpm. The resulting suspension was passed through 8 layers of sterile gauze to remove stroma and large clumps of cells. The filtrate contained 100,000 cells per cubic millimeter. The suspension was concentrated to 1,000,00 cells per cubic millimeter, then serially diluted with saline to concentrations of 500,000, 250,000, 125.000,

62,500, 31,250 and 15,625 cells per cubic millimeter. One-half ml.
of an even suspension of each dilution was then inoculated subcutaneously in groups of 3 mice.

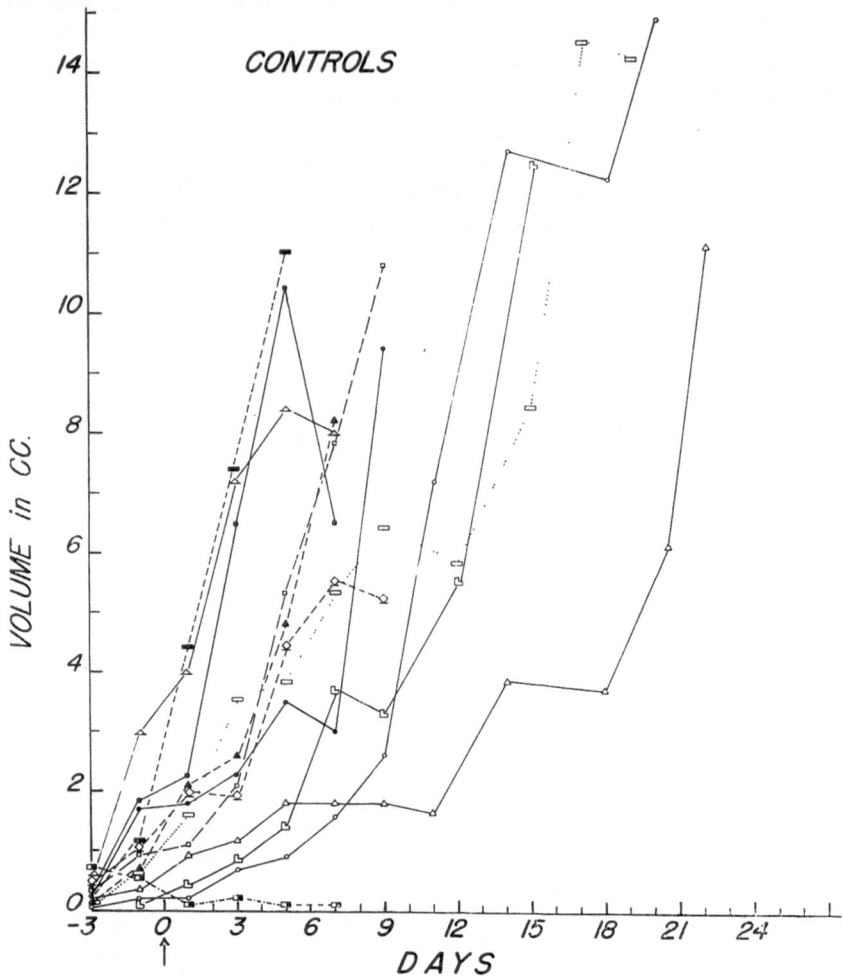

Fig. 2. Chart showing growth rate curves of ependymomas growing subcutaneously. The volume
of the tumor is shown on the ordinate, days after transplantation (at — 3) on the abscissa.
Each line represents the repeated measurements of the tumor in 1 mouse. Note the variability
in growth rates. One transplant failed to grow. (This figure is reproduced through the courtesy
of the editor of The American Journal of Roentgenology, Radium Therapy and Nuclear Medicine.)

The resulting growths were difficult to explain quantitatively.
Weak dilutions grew before high concentrations of cells. The same
dilution grew in a few days in 1 mouse, in a few weeks in a littermate and not at all in the third littermate. It is assumed that the

suspension of cells delivered to the animals was homogenous, hence the conclusion is reached that even in genetically pure populations, individual resistance to neoplasia is still present.

These factors of individual resistance are present in different organs of the body in the same animal. This feature was demonstrated when 0.2 ml. of the previously described homogenate (50,000 cells per cubic millimeter) was injected in the tail vein of ten A albino mice. The results are shown in table 1. The possible fates of a homogenous suspension of glial cells therefore are:

1. Cells may die.
2. Cells may leave veins in pelvis and grow locally.
3. Cells may enter right side of circulation and grow in lung.
4. Cells may pass pulmonary vascular bed and grow in other organs.

The "soil" in which gliomas grow may be any organ of the body, but it is not known why tumor cells grow widely in one animal, and not at all in another. The mechanisms of individual and organ resistances to growth of tumors have been investigated but little.

6. *External factors affect the growth and appearance of gliomas.* Comment has already been made that tumors in general grow more rapidly when subcutaneous transplants are made from saline suspensions of cells than from solid pieces. *Cohn* and *Zimmerman* (1955) found that an ependymoma derived from subcutaneous transplants in the mouse became amorphous in the allantoic membrane of the chick egg, then re-acquired an ependymal appearance when returned to the subcutaneous tissue of the mouse. These observations will not surprise pathologists who have studied the same neoplasm in different locations, e. g., a metastatic carcinoma of the breast growing in the brain may contain cuboidal or columnar cells arranged in acini, but in the cerebral dura the same cells may be compressed by the connective tissue and become spindle shaped or lose the glandular pattern. Similarly, glial cells with the shape of a carrot *in situ* may become round when suspended in saline.

Roentgen rays have striking effects upon gliomas even when given in single doses. Rate of growth of an experimental ependymal tumor was not affected by single doses of 200 or 400 r., although transient histologic alterations occured. It is of interest to note that the limited preliminary experiments (*Netsky* and coll., 1952) showed a stimulating effect of 400 r. and have been widely quoted, but the definitive experiments (*Netsky* and coll., 1956) have been largely ignored on this matter. It is safe to say that evidence is lacking for a growth stimulating effect of low doses of radiation. Doses of

1200 r. caused a transient depression of growth. Large doses of 3000 or 5000 r. destroyed the tumor *if all the cells received the radiation*. Evidence was presented that if some cells were not exposed to the full dose, the tumor might regrow even more rapidly than normally. The total growth curve of the tumor was then "diphasic".

The supporting data in part included experiments in which 3000 r. was delivered to the tumor in a glass dish; the radiated mass, known to have received the full dose, then was transplanted subcutaneously and failed to grow. These experiments showed that 3000 r. was completely destructive for this experimental glioma, and that neither radiation of the tumor bed nor changes in the surrounding blood vessels were necessary for lethal effects. The only growth-stimulating effect of x-rays in these experiments occurred in the second part of the diphasic curve 8 to 15 days after radiation. The histologic effects of x-rays are discussed in section 9.

7. *Experimental gliomas tend to become ependymal or unclassifiable in successive transplants.* It was stated by *Zimmerman* and *Maier* (1948/49) that from a single primary glioma it was possible to grow subcutaneously two or more different "pure" tumors and later that the tumors were morphologically constant in over 100 serial transplants. *Perese* and *Moore* (1960) were able to grow ependymona in many successive generations of transplants, but could not maintain astrocytic or oligodendroglial tumors, noting an ependymomatous appearance after the tenth generation of transplantation. My experience is more in accord with the latter authors, except that I found some tumors ultimately became unclassifiable, and designated these as undifferentiated gliomas.

Perese and *Moore* (1960) also discussed the change of glioblastoma multiforme into sarcoma with successive transplants. This observation is probably best explained as an initial induction of both glioblastoma and sarcoma, and the continued growth and outstripping of the glial cells by the connective tissue tumor. Their observation is confirmed that it is difficult to maintain the appearance of glioblastoma multiforme after many generations of transplantation. This tumor is composed of various cell types, and some cells overgrow others.

8. *"Pure" tumors probably do not exist.* The implication of a "pure" tumor is that a uniform cell population is present. The majority of human brain tumors and of induced experimental gliomas are mixed — in the sense that many different glial cell types may be recognized in them. In general, tumors are usually named as if they were pure — astrocytoma, ependymoma, etc. But this unitary diagnosis of astrocytoma may still be made when other cells are

seen within the tumor. The obligation felt by the pathologist to make a single diagnosis often results in ignoring some histologic features. It is known that these induced tumors may be divided, and one or another element grow out in the different transplants. From a single brain tumor, two or more morphologically different tumors may grow, although as indicated previously, the differences may not be maintained in generations of successive transplants. Reversion to ependymal or unclassifiable glioma, or more rapid growth of fibrous connective tissue elements may occur in the process of multiple transplantation.

9. *Glial cells may be multi-potential in neoplasia.* The capacity of oligodendroglial cells to become astrocytic has been noted in reparative efforts (*Koenig* and coll., 1961). The evidence for ready interchange of these two cell types in neoplasms was discussed by *Cooper* (1935). An even more diverse change is suggested by transplantation experiments. Astrocytomas made to grow rapidly by early transplantation may become spongioblastic in appearance. The reverse may occur when growth is slowed by delaying the time of transplantation until the tumor has reached very large size. In this way the astrocyte is as much precursor of the spongioblast as the usually expressed embryologic consideration that spongioblasts precede astrocytes. The appearance of the cell is related to its *rate* of growth under these conditions.

Astrocytes growing in compressed zones also may become spongioblastic; appearance then is related to *site* of growth. The artificial lines between glial tumor cell types are man-made, and the relation of tumor cells to embryonic cells has little support. The equally arbitrary subdivisions between gliomas are being recognized with increasing clarity. *Willis* (1948) has rightly insisted that the types of gliomas are not sharply distinct — "unfortunately . . . once we have given a name to . . . an arbitrarily determined group, we are apt to forget its arbitrary character and to accept the name as denoting a specific entity." The value of the modified Bailey-Cushing classification used throughout this paper is mainly for purposes of description.

10. *Histologic appearance often correlates poorly with biologic behavior.* A frequently expressed aim of the pathologist dealing with brain tumors is to correlate histologic appearance with biologic behavior (e. g. *Zülch*, 1957). These biologic features include prognosis, capacity to metastasize, location, ease of excision, and response to radiation. To achieve this aim, however, it is necessary to deal with large groups and ignore individual cases. For example, a medulloblastoma in the cerebellum of one child may melt away

under the influence of x-rays, but the same tumor in another child, causing comparable clinical signs and having the same morphologic appearance, may not respond at all to radiation. These tumors are histologically similar but strikingly different in at least one biologic response. Glioblastoma multiforme usually is a rapidly evolving tumor causing death within a year, but histologically comparable tumors are compatible with a survival period as long as 14 years (*Netsky* and coll., 1950). The pathologist offering an opinion as to radiosensitivity or pontifically prognosticating gives suppositions of statistical rather than individual significance.

The discrepancy between histologic appearance and biologic behavior was notable in our study of the effects of radiation on experimental gliomas (*Netsky* and coll., 1956). The wide range of growth patterns of the unirradiated controls has already been noted. Yet whether the ependymoma doubled in size every two days or slowly enlarged for two weeks, its morphologic appearance was remarkably constant. Radiation caused definite histologic changes described in detail in our publication, but unless the tumor was completely destroyed, the cellular changes decreased and soon disappeared with lapse of time. Tumors having extraordinarily rapid regrowth after initial inhibition ("diphasic growth") still were morphologically similar to slow growing controls. As stated previously, (*Netsky* and coll., 1956) "the microscopic appearance was a poor means of judging what had happened in the past or was occuring presently in the neoplasm". To this should be added "and is equally inferior for determining the future of the tumor or its host". It is clear that better tools are needed to measure biologic alterations of these tumors.

The last problem to be considered is to what extent the tumor of mouse is comparable to that of man. Histologic similarity is not sufficient to allow us to say that these tumors are biologically the same, or that they will respond similarly to therapy. It is fairly well established in human material, as already noted, that histologically similar tumors differ in their response to radiation therapy. It is obvious that unknown factors of resistance are present in man as in mouse. It seems probable that the study of resistance — of the individual tumor, organ, host or species — may lead to significant answers to our knowledge of these tumors and their treatment.

Summary

The induction and transplantation of gliomas is considered critically under the following headings:

1. Species and strain of animal are important factors in the induction of experimental brain tumors; genetic factors play a role in determining the incidence of gliomas.

2. Individual resistance to induction of brain tumors occurs under identical conditions.

3. The site of implantation is a partial determinant of the type of glioma induced; the cells exposed to the carcinogen are a factor in determining which neoplasm is produced.

4. Local tissue resistance to growth of gliomas is low; failure of these tumors to grow extra-cerebrally is not dependent upon the "soil".

5. Despite low tissue resistance, the rate of growth of gliomas under controlled conditions is extremely variable; unknown growth factors exist in the tumor or in the host.

6. External factors affect growth and appearance of gliomas.

7. Experimental gliomas tend to become ependymal or unclassifiable in successive transplants.

8. "Pure" glial tumors probably do not exist.

9. Glial cells may be multi-potential in neoplasia.

10. Histologic appearance often correlates poorly with biologic behavior.

References

Cohn, A., and *H. M. Zimmerman,* Growth behavior of chemically induced mouse brain tumors in the chick embryo. Excerpta med., sec. 8, *8* (1955), 818 (abstract). — *Cooper, E. R. A.,* The relation of oligocytes and astrocytes in cerebral tumors. J. Path. Bact. *41* (1935), 259—266. — *Ewing, J.,* Neoplastic diseases. Saunders, Philadelphia, 1940. — *Koenig, H., M. Bunge* and *R. Bunge,* Personal communication. 1961. — *Netsky, M. G., B. August* and *W. Fowler,* The longevity of patients with glioblastoma multiforme. J. Neurosurg., Springfield, 7 (1950), 261—269. — *Netsky, M. G., J. R. Freid, B. Corsentino* and *H. M. Zimmerman,* The effect of single doses of x-ray on an experimentally induced glioma. J. Neuropath., Baltimore, *11* (1952), 87—88. — *Netsky, M. G., J. Shapiro, M. Hoffman, B. Corsentino, J. R. Freid* and *H. M. Zimmerman,* The effects of single doses of roentgen radiation on experimentally induced gliomas: with a critical review of the effects of roentgen radiation on gliomas in man. Amer. J. Roentgenol. *76* (1956), 351—366. — *Perese, D. M.,* and *G. E. Moore,* Methods of induction and histogenesis of experimental brain tumors. J. Neurosurg., Springfield, *17* (1960), 677—699. — *Willis, R. A.,* Pathology of tumors. Mosby, St. Louis, 1948. — *Zimmerman, H. M.,* and *H. Arnold,* Chemical carcinogens and animal species as factors in experimental brain tumors. J. Neuropath., Baltimore, 2 (1943), 416 to 417. — *Zimmerman, H. M.,* and *H. Arnold,* Experimental brain tumors. IV. The incidence in different strains of mice. Cancer Res. *4* (1944), 98—101. — *Zimmerman, H. M.,* and *N. Maier,* Experimental brain tumors. Proc. N. Y. Path. Soc. (1948/49), 40—42. — *Zülch, K. J.,* Brain tumors: their biology and pathology. Springer. New York, 1957.

Discussion

Dr. Zülch: Dr. Netsky, I thank you very much for your report which contains a condensed accumulation of facts that really need a full afternoon's discussion. There are so many problems which you have touched that each of them should be discussed separately. One thing I may just say at the end of this opening of the discussion. If we had not known that you had a Janus head, that is if we had not had so many valuable contributors to a simple classification this forenoon, it would have been very difficult to base any morphological classification on your observations. They are of course correct, but they make us think and discuss and argue again. They are naturally very specialised and have no bearing on the routine classification which is simply an aid to the clinician. But I think this paper is so full of new points of view and observations that we should start the discussion. Would you begin with the discussion or shall we first have Dr. Schiefer's paper? . . .

Then I ask you, Dr. Schiefer to read your paper.

Morphology of Experimental Brain Tumours

By

B. Schiefer

With 8 Figures

The experimental production of tumours with chemical agents is quite different from the normal spontaneous development of a tumour but by this method it is possible to imitate experimentally the development of normal cellular units into tumours. The findings of

Table 1

A	*Tumours of Neuroepithelial origin:*	
	Medulloblastoma	1
	Oligodendroglioma	4
	Glioblastoma multiforme	6
	Astrocytoma	1
	Ependymoma	1
B	*Tumours of Mesenchymal origin:*	
	Retothelial sarcomas	2
	Sarcomas (Fibrosarcoma, Polymorph cell sarcoma)	23
C	*Tumours of doubtful origin:*	
	Probably mesenchymal	2

$$= 26\cdot4\ ^\circ/_\circ \left(\begin{array}{c} 40\ \text{out} \\ \text{of}\ 151 \end{array} \right)$$

Zimmerman and *Arnold* (1941) and also *Seligman* and *Shear* (1939) are very interesting and important, but study of the microphotograms of the investigations of these authors raised many doubts as to diagnosis. For this reason we have carried out our own investigations using the pellet technique with 20-methylcholanthrene (see also *Schiefer*, 1959).

Amongst the 151 brains of mice which reached the tumour-bearing age (that is those animals which died after the 65th day, the day after the first mesodermal tumour appeared) were 13 tumours of neuroglial origin, 25 tumours from the mesoderm and 2 tumours with a doubtful diagnosis (see table1). The experiments were performed on normal mice without susceptibility to tumours.

The diagnosis was established according to the classification of *Zülch* (1956 a and 1956 b).

Description

1. Medulloblastoma.

In the cerebellum there is a group of cells which are larger than the granular cells. The nuclei are very dark, oval or turnip-shaped, the cytoplasm is scanty, many mitotic figures are seen in the tumour and occasionally there are pseudorosettes (Fig. 1).

2. Oligodendroglioma.

In a fine fibrous network there are small dark isomorphic cells (Fig. 2). The network is like a honeycomb. There is only a small amount of stroma. Many mitotic figures are seen. At the edge occasionally the tumour cells surround ganglion cells (Fig. 3).

3. Glioblastoma multiforme.

Beside the tumours first described, there are 6 other tumours originally of glial nature, where we find a part of the tumour with small cells and another part with long and polygonal cells (Fig. 4) in the vicinity of the blood vessels with positive reticulin staining in most cases. There is also a group of cells, evolving towards monster cells (Fig. 5). In the middle of these cells there are often small vessels.

4. Astrocytoma.

In the neighbourhood of the ventricle there is a network with the structure of a honeycomb in which the nuclei are seen as small dark balls. With higher magnification you see a cytoplasm with radiating processes which form a network. There is a commencing muco-degeneration (Fig. 6).

5. Ependymoma.

In the left ventricle there is an anisomorphic tumour with cells with scanty cytoplasm and chromatin rich nuclei. There is no stroma. It is possible to call this an ependymoma-like tumour and it resembles the variant of an ependymoma of the foramen of Monro described by *Zülch* (Fig. 233 in: *Zülch*, 1956 b).

6. Mesodermal tumors.

There were 23 mesodermal tumours resembling fibrosarcomas or polymorphcellular sarcomas and 2 resembling retothelial sarcomas. It is very important to note, that these tumours have begun to grow purely mesodermally without glial components.

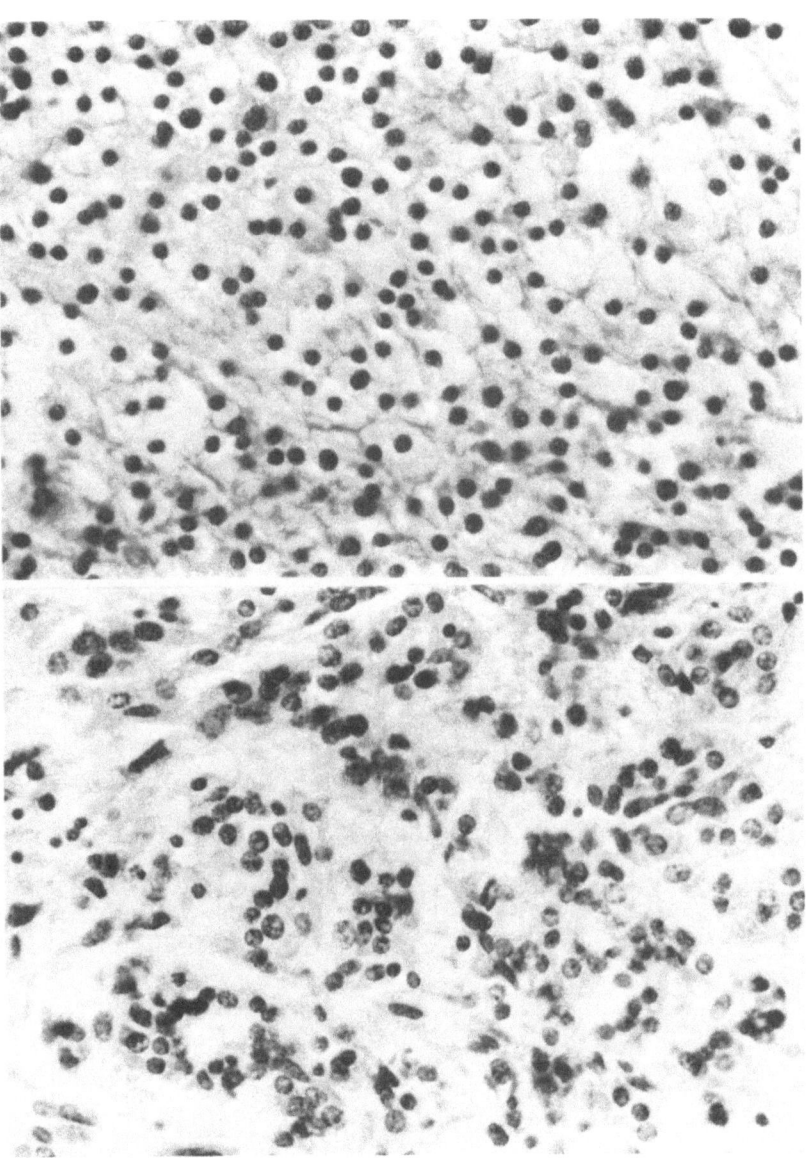

Fig. 1.

Fig. 2.

Fig. 1. Medulloblastoma: oval or turnip shaped cells and occasionally pseudorosettes (90), HE, 400 ×.

Fig. 2. Oligodendroglioma: "Honeycomb" structure (89), HE, 400 ×.

7. Doubtful cases.

In two cases it was impossible to establish an exact diagnosis. Both tumours are characterised by large nuclei with a sharp chromatin structure without cytoplasm. There are many mitotic figures. The silver staining was negative. It is possible to compare these

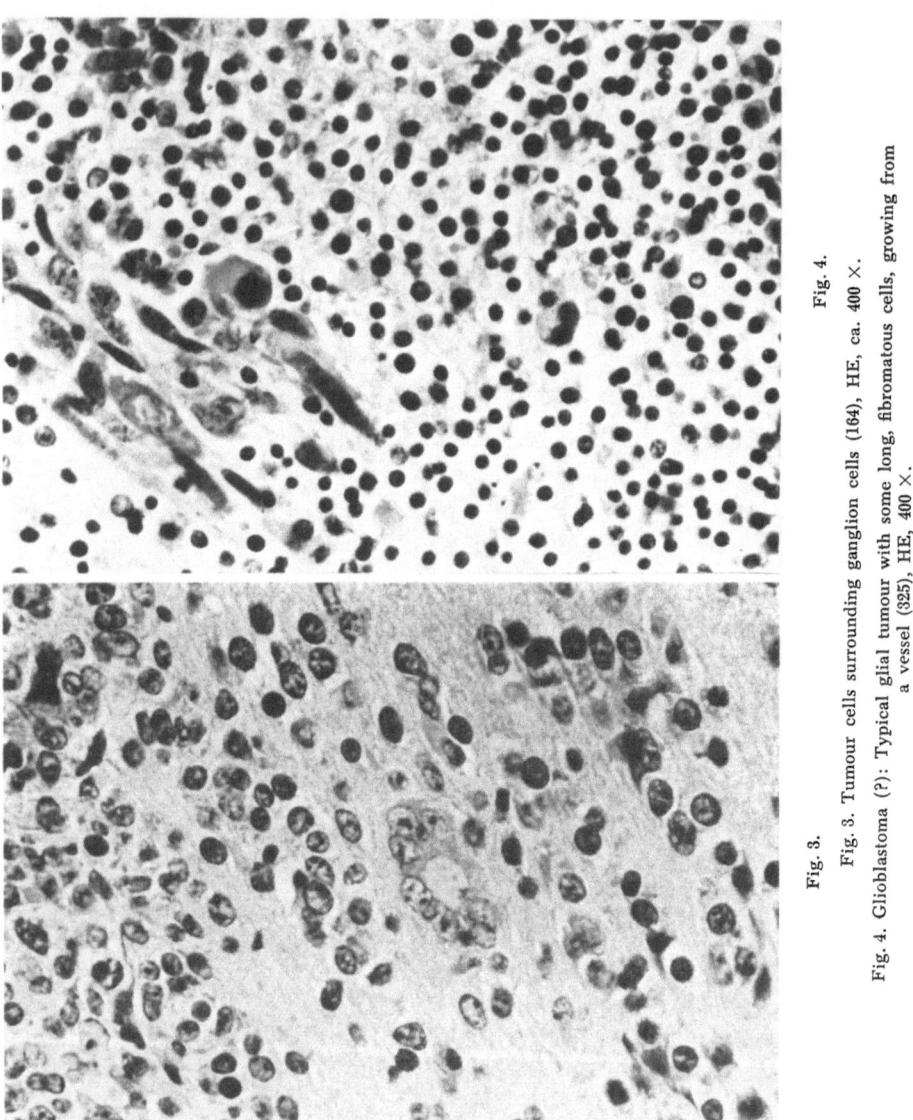

Fig. 3.

Fig. 3. Tumour cells surrounding ganglion cells (164), HE, ca. 400 ×.

Fig. 4.

Fig. 4. Glioblastoma (?): Typical glial tumour with some long, fibromatous cells, growing from a vessel (325), HE, 400 ×.

tumours with a spontaneous case in a dog (709/58), described by us *(Dahme-Schiefer)* in 1960, as an afibrillar retothelial tumour.

8. Epithelial neoplasms.

Epithelial tumours which we saw in some cases in our first series might be explained as epithelial cells were displaced by the operation. They are therefore only briefly mentioned.

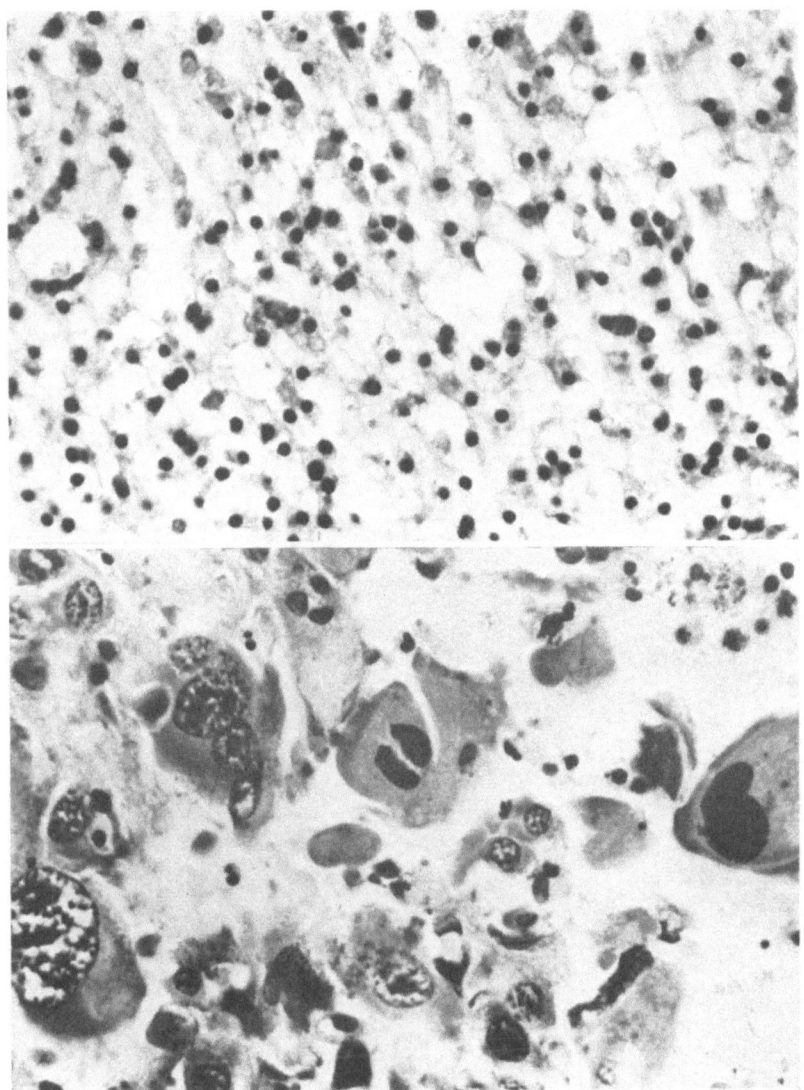

Fig. 6.

Fig. 6. Astrocytoma (332), HE, 400 ×.

Fig. 5.

Fig. 5. Monster cells which developed from the mesodermal cells (325), HE, 400 ×.

Discussion

Two points are important in my opinion:

First:

In spite of the fact that typical pure tumours developed, we see that all the experimental tumours are characterised by irregularity of the cells, many mitotic figures and a reaction of the stroma in-

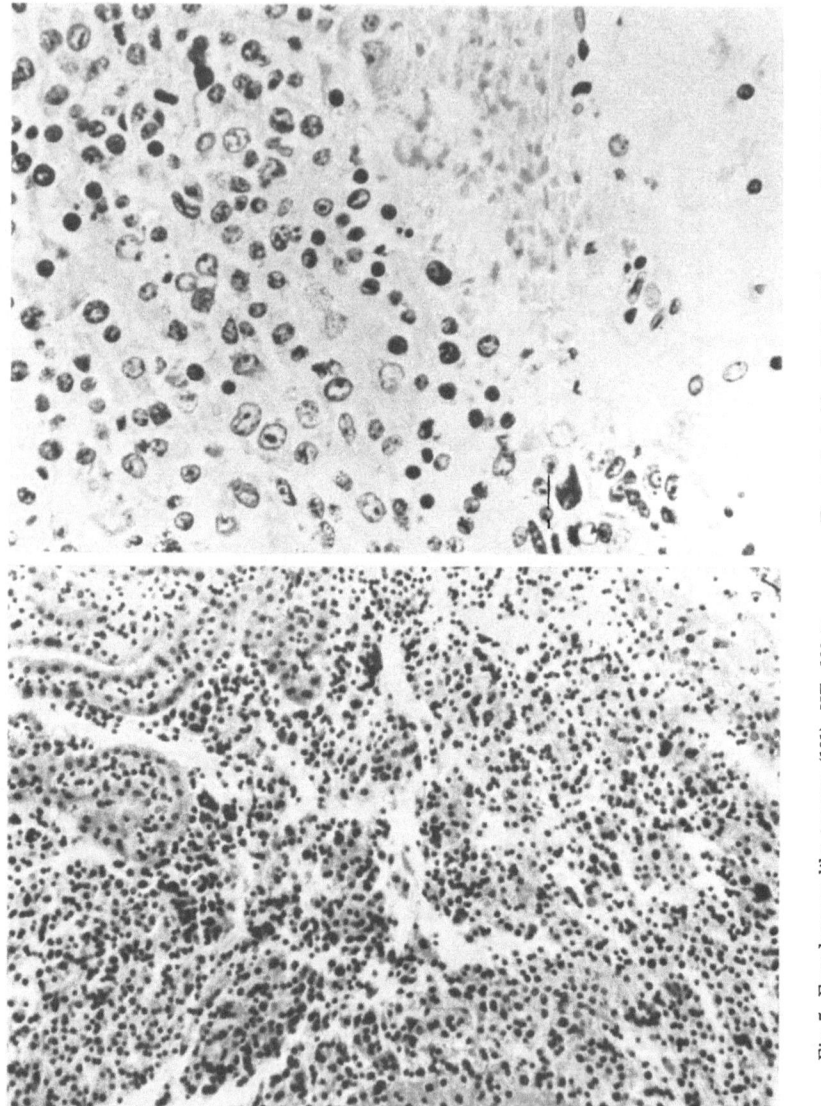

Fig. 8. Probably afibrillar RS-sarcoma (147), HE, 400 ×.

Fig. 7. Ependymoma-like tumour (191), HE, 100 ×.

dicating a malignant tendency. We see the same in the spontaneous brain tumours of animals.

The second point is a question:

Does irritation by a neoplastic tissue induce tumour growth in a second part of the tissue? *Feigin* and *Gross* described 3 cases of glioblastoma multiforme in which the vessels developed into sarcomas. We see in our cases that the large tumour cells are growing from the vessel walls, and therefore we believe, that they are of mesodermal origin. There is still the problem as to whether the two components are induced by the same carcinogenic action or if the glial tumour induced a secondary growth of the mesenchymal element.

When *Zimmerman* and *Arnold* and also *Netsky* say that within certain limits the site of pellet implantation determines the character of the developing tumour it is necessary to emphasize the limitations of this statement: it is not possible to say that only the mother cells of the tumours come under the influence of the carcinogen. It is still a moot point why in one case a mixed tumour with neuroglial and mesodermal elements develops, whereas in another case only the neuroglial or the mesodermal element is showing tumour growth. It seems therefore to be necessary to make further investigations in which the very commencement of the developing tumours can be made visible.

Literature

Dahme, E., and *B. Schiefer*, Intracranielle Geschwülste bei Tieren. Zbl. Vet. med. *VII* (1960), 341—363. — *Feigin, I. H.*, and *S. W. Gross*, Sarcoma arising in glioblastoma of the brain. Amer. J. Path. *XXXI* (1955), 633—653. — *Schiefer, B..* Über die experimentelle Erzeugung von Gehirntumoren mit Methylcholantren. Zbl. Neurochir. *XVIII* (1958), 360—373. — *Seligman, A. M.*, and *M. G. Shear*, Experimental production of brain tumours in mice with methylcholanthrene. Amer. J. Cancer *XXXVII* (1939), 364—395. — *Zimmerman, H. M.*, and *H. Arnold*, Experimental brain tumours. Cancer Res. *I* (1941), 919—924. — *Zülch, K. J.*, Die Hirngeschwülste in biologischer und morphologischer Darstellung. 2. Aufl., J. A. Barth, Leipzig, 1956 a. — *Idem*, in: Olivecrona-Tönnis, Handb. d. Neurochirurgie, III. Bd., Springer, Berlin-Göttingen-Heidelberg, 1956 b.

Discussion

Dr. Zülch: Thank you, Dr. Schiefer. Both papers are open to discussion. Would anyone like to comment on this?

Dr. Hamperl: I would point out that in regard to these experimental brain tumours we are sometimes in the same position as we are in regard to human tumours. There also occur mixtures of human tumours at other sites. For example adeno-carcinoma of the stomach or the breast which sometimes grow like a scirrhus, but on the other hand can produce mucus and we are sometimes in difficulty as to the classification of this tumour. In general pathology the principle adopted was formulated long ago by Kauffmann, when he said: a potiori fit denominatio. One should designate a tumour according to its greater part or dominant feature or the differentiation which occurs in its tissue. We know that besides this differentiation which is the basis for the name which we give to such a tumour there may occur other differentiations. Thus you have said — and I am in complete agreement with you — that there is often a mixture of cell types and that we should not be troubled too much by this because probably in most cases we are able to say which family of cells in the mixture is the privileged one and to this we should stick and derive the name

The next point I would make is about what you call transitions. As a histologist I don't like the transition from one fully differentiated cell into another fully differentiated cell, because general pathology again has shown that these transitions mostly occur by the evolution of a strain of undifferentiated cells and then these undifferentiated cells undergo differentiation in different directions. So I would not say that a cell which has once differentiated in one direction changes its differentiation into another highly differentiated cell, but that probably in the host of cells you produced there are some that have all the potentialities of development and differentiation along other lines as well. We call this indirect metaplasia and we are strongly against all attempts to establish a direct metaplasia. These were the two remarks I had to make.

Dr. Zülch: Thank you, Dr. Hamperl. Dr. Netsky, would you like to answer?

Dr. Netsky: I think, we have one problem that many neuropathologists have to face, the group will I think confirm that we often use the dominant feature in the diagnostic method whereby we give a single name, but it is also true that many neuropathologists feel an obligation to a clinician and often give a prognostic diagnosis, so that for instance if one has predominantly astrocytes but sees a few fields of endothelial hyperplasia and foci of necroses with a little pseudo-palisading, these features may make us diagnose glioblastoma multiforme, even though it is everywhere else astrocytoma. We really have never settled this, sometimes we tend to one or to the other, and it may possibly he a source of confusion. I think we should probably stick to a general principle but we usually do not. With regard to the question of transition I can only say it is a proposition I was taught in general pathology but it must be reexamined. I think much of the evidence has been based on a static study of tumours that are in one stage as one usually sees in histological preparations. The new views we are getting from tissue culture and other dynamic methods are giving us new insight. My purpose was not to explode this idea completely and say that it is no longer valuable, but we must think of the possibility of major transitions and of cells developing in various directions. May we think about it and not say this is the final conclusion?

Dr. Rubinstein: Dr. Netsky has just raised an important point for the diagnostic pathologist. We have discussed the question of calling a tumour by its major component, but there is a strong feeling, and I think it is justified, that for the pathologist's diagnosis it is necessary to emphasize the most malignant part of the tumour. And if you find as in the case just described an astrocytoma where there is a small focus of glioblastoma, what is the responsibility of the pathologist? I think many would accept the principle that we must call this a glioblastoma, i. e. the principle is that you report on the most malignant part of the tumour.

Dr. Zülch: Why shouldn't you say an astrocytoma with development or transition to glioblastoma which will probably be more correct? These cases have a longer survival period than the primary glioblastoma. There is one point I would like to menätion. I frankly admit that human tumours are mixed and it is not to be thought that nature would make an experiment such as are made in tissue culture, but one thing which often was forgotten in the first days of brain tumour classification is that we have to look at a tumour which has invaded brain tissue. And if you look at Bailey's first descriptions of a medulloblastoma you will find definite cerebellar astrocytes, definite ganglion cells of the cerebellum, definite granular cells of the tissue which has been invaded. And if we find astrocytes and oligocytes — and we have done just that in the last few days to make sure and we come back to this in the discussion on the oligodendrogliomas — the prevalence of oligodendroglioma cells for instance in a glioblastoma is not surprising. You see then we found that even in a glioblastoma there are quite a number of oligodendroglia cells, but these are normal, they are just looking like normal oligodendroglial cells with regressive changes. So I think we should never forget that what we examine is often a piece of the brain which has been invaded, where we can show the myelin sheaths very easily and oligodendroglial cells, axons, ganglion cells and so on. This we have to bear in mind, particularly in cerebellar tumours.

Dr. Netsky: This is certainly true when one examines clinical material. But it is different when one has experimental material and can subdivide it and grow out different kinds of tumours and one has unequivocal evidence of the capacity of this material to differentiate. The problem is whether you are sure that you can define a normal cell.

Dr. Kersting: Are you sure that a normal cell will survive after transplantation?

Dr. Netsky: I have made that assumption and I admit it is an assumption. We are making many assumptions here which are taken as absolute truth, but require investigation. My assumption is that the normal cell will not continue to grow autonomously in transplantation.

Dr. Woolf: You described one experiment in which you had an experimental glioma with a certain histological picture, then you irradiated it and there were temporary changes in the histology and then it reverted to the same appearance as before. And then I thought you said that in spite of the fact that the growth has been speeded up it has the same histological appearance. Can you tell me if I have got that correct and how it fits in with what you said earlier that radiation does not cause an increase of growth. It is obviously very important.

Dr. Netsky: I am sorry I had a limited amount of time and therefore had to condense a great deal of material. The contention was that very low doses of radiation have no growth stimulating effect. This I am certain of although it has been stated otherwise as a result of our initial experiments. With bigger doses stimulation of growth may occur, particularly when a tumour has received what ostensibly is a lethal dose, but certain cells outside the radiated zone have received only partial amounts of this. These latter cells may then be stimulated to further growth. It may in part be caused by substances arising in the destroyed tumour and there may be other factors. This is the only circumstance in which there is acceleration of growth by X-rays — partial radiation.

Dr. Ringertz: May I continue this discussion by pointing out the phenomenon known to the ordinary tumour biologist, that there is an enhancement of transplantable growth when the cells concerned are mixed with incompatible cells? If you transplant a mixture of tumour cells in the subcutis of mice containing incompatible cells with very small doses of compatible ones of the same kind, you will find that the very small dose of compatible cells grows out much more rapidly than if you had put them in pure dose. And the same occurs if you begin radiating in vitro parts of a tumour suspension and then put a small dose of non-radiated cells into the mixture and introduce them into the animal. The enhancement is caused by the presence of the irradiated cells. And this fits very well with your experiments that a tumour which is mostly but not quite radiated to destruction is very dangerous because the rest of it grows rapidly.

Dr. Zülch: Thank you, Dr. Ringertz.

Dr. Netsky: Yes, there are numerous other observations of a comparable sort, for instance the radiation of yeast cells. If these cells are mixed with normal yeast cells the normal yeast cells may grow rapidly. So when radiation damage occurs and these radiation damaged cells are largely intermixed with normal cells or neoplastic cells they may then accelerate growth. This I think is well supported by many types of observations including yeasts and these observations of yours.

Dr. Zülch: Any other contributions, comments, criticism? Dr. Calvo.

Dr. Calvo: I would like to know Dr. Schiefer if there is reticulin in the experimental tumours surrounding those giant cells or whether they may be oligodendrocytes that have become giant.

Dr. Schiefer: The reticulum staining shows reticulin only in the parts where there are giant cells, i. e. around vessels. In the other parts it is a pure neuroepithelial tumour without tissue from the reticulum.

Dr. Zülch: Dr. Schiefer did not mention, I think, that what he showed was a monstrocellular sarcoma within a mixed glioma. We have seen that frequently. I wonder if you did not see that frequently.

Dr. Netsky: I am not certain that I know what a monstrocellular sarcoma is.

Dr. Zülch: I am sorry, but you have seen what we have shown, perhaps you would comment on the question as to whether you have seen strains of giant and monstrous cells like those in our tumours.

Dr. Netsky: There is no doubt that I have seen them, but whether we should be calling them monstrocellular sarcoma is the issue.

Dr. Zülch: Well, I agree, the question is, if we call those parts blastoma and other parts not, when the blastoma part consisted of about one third of the cells very often.

Dr. Rubinstein: Dr. Schiefer projected two pictures that illustrate his point. In the first one there were some giant cells around the blood vessels. Of course I think we have to debate here whether the finding of giant cells around blood vessels necessarily means they have arisen from the blood vessel wall. This to me is not clearly established. The second point concerns the second picture which showed a glioma with one large cell in the middle of it. It seems to me that we have to discuss here whether the single large cell is really a sarcoma cell in the middle of a lot of glioma.

Dr. Schiefer: This photo was taken in the neighbourhood of great tumour cells. It is only in this photo that it appears to be in the neuroglial part.

Dr. Zülch: This raises the question as to whether any giant cell is a sarcoma cell and I think we would not go as far as that. You see, this giant cell part here is definitely a strand of thick connective tissue. We will get the slides out for you and on the right hand side you will find a huge part of the tumour looking like this monstrocellular tissue and on the left side you see the gliogenic tumour which looks like an oligodendroglioma in a glioblastoma multiforme.

Dr. Rubinstein: Could we see the next picture? Yes.

Dr. Schiefer: It is from a spontaneous glioblastoma of a dog. There are many different points in this tumour, there are spindle cell parts and other parts with large vessel proliferation and round cell parts, and this is from a large cell part with one giant cell in the neighbourhood of ...

Dr. Rubinstein: Could not this be just a giant glial cell, one single cell in the middle of a glioma?

Dr. Schiefer: Yes, in a glioma, in a glioblastoma.

Dr. Rubinstein: Why then a cell of a different nature? Why not a glial cell?

Dr. Zülch: Did you really think that it was a mesodermal cell?

Dr. Schiefer: It is because nowhere in the tumour are there giant cells except around the vessels. It is often like this.

Dr. Zülch: Do you understand? He said that the giant cells are almost restricted to the neighbourhood of the vessels·even in this particular case which is a spontaneous tumour in a dog, in a boxer.

Dr. Rubinstein: I wonder how many people would be convinced that a case has been made out that the single cell there is quite different from the rest of the tumour.

Dr. Schiefer: It is a question as to whether the cell is derived from the vessel wall, but I think it is hard to say because this is an experimental tumour.

Dr. Rubinstein: Here again you see a giant cell in the region of a blood vessel and I agree that this relationship is there, but if you distinguish observation from deduction, you are deducing that in this case it arises from the blood vessel wall, but what I see here is a large tumour cell in the region of a blood vessel. I think it is crucial to decide whether this cell is in fact a glial cell near a blood vessel or a sarcoma cell arising in the blood vessel wall.

Dr. Zülch: I think you could not deduce that from this particular section. I mean, would you be convinced by the first, the large one which we have seen?

Dr. Rubinstein: I would like to see the section.

Dr. Netsky: It is always a cautious answer to insist on seeing sections, if not, then special stains.

Dr. Zülch: Well, I thank you both again, Dr. Netsky and Dr. Schiefer for your contributions and we proceed now to Dr. Kersting who will give his observations on the tissue culture of human brain tumours.

4. Tissue Culture

Tissue Culture and the Classification of Brain Tumours

By

G. Kersting*

Our contribution today on "Tissue Culture and the Classification of Brain Tumours" covers only a few general aspects of a very complicated problem. All technical details are omitted and questions of specific interest will be discussed later in relation to the subjects of the later sessions. All the statements that follow are based exclusively on our own experimental investigations including tissue cultures of about 500 cerebral neoplasms which seems to be the largest series so far.

Two fundamental questions have to be answered before any further discussion of tissue culture and classification problems is justifiable:

1. Whether results obtained by extracorporeal cultivation can be transferred to *in situ* conditions,

2. whether a cytogenetic classification of the neuroectodermal neoplasms adequately corresponds to the given facts.

Let us start with the second:

The classification of gliomas proposed by *Bailey* and *Cushing,* and modified by *Zülch* and coll., although conceived on a "histogenetic basis" is not a histogenetic classification in the meaning of general pathology. In general pathology "histogenetic" means a classification of tumours according to the tissues, from which they originate. For every tissue — a tumour. In this sense the cited classification of brain tumours has to be regarded as cytogenetic or cytological. Morphological diagnosis depends on the species of the prevailing cells, as one regards them as the origin or matrix of the given individual blastoma. Critics of this classification have suggested that brain tumours should be classified as the blastomas of other organs according to the tissue, and that for a more detailed and specialized diagnosis one should not look for cytological details but for histo-

---

* See: *Kersting, G.,* Die Gewebszüchtung menschlicher Hirngeschwülste. Springer-Verlag, Berlin-Göttingen-Heidelberg, 1961.

logical characteristics such as mode of distribution, regional differences, participation of mesenchyma and so on.

This broadly outlined problem — the histogenetic or cytogenetic origin and classification of brain tumours — became more interesting, when tissue culture experiments demonstrated that by this means certain features of the problem could be isolated and directly examined.

The specialized research in brain tumour pathology has not so far been able to produce a convincing theory of the etiology and formal genesis of neuroectodermal blastomas. Most investigators only try to adapt the various theories of general pathology to the specific conditions of the central nervous system, assuming that fundamental differences between general and neural pathology in this field need not be expected.

There can be no real doubt that these theories, especially the field theory of *Willis* which regards as the origin of every blastoma the initial transformation of a whole area of cells — the field — strongly favours the concept of a histological or histogenetic classification. If the tumour producing process starts with a transformation of tissues, then a histological consideration seems certainly to be more adequate. This is even more the case when we learn from the experiments of Drs. *Zimmerman, Netsky* and coll., that the intracerebral implantation of cancerogenous substances in mice leads to the production of mixed gliomas with regional differences. Experimentally induced mouse gliomas are said to show ependymoma-like structures near the ventricles, astrocytic portions within the deep white matter and oligodendroglial elements prevail in the cortical and subcortical regions.

Human glioblastomas show similar differences and a great variety of structure. The various parts of a human glioblastoma may be so different, that doubts as to its identity arise. Following the histogenetic concept, that the structural configuration of a given glioblastoma is the natural consequence of its origin from heteromorphous sources, one had to conclude, that after the explantation of minute particles of 20, 50 or 100 single cells from different parts of the blastoma the colonies formed *in vitro* ought to show a correspondingly divergent cellular composition. In the case of experimentally induced mouse gliomas such a development into different directions really seems to take place. After ex- and transplantation of the mixed gliomas the cellular composition of emerging daughter colonies more or less strictly follows the regional structure of the original blastoma. The primary mixed glioma develops into different cellularly homogenous daughter neoplasms.

Human glioblastomas behave quite differently. The 80—120 in vitro cultures of a single glioblastoma multiforme are — as far as cellular composition and histological structure are concerned — exactly the same. Cellular homogeneity is rarely found and only under certain conditions (in a subgroup of fusiform glioblastoma and in the cerebral glioblastoma of children). But in a series of 120 glioblastomas we have never observed that some cultures from a particular tumour show an astrocytic, others a giant cell, and a third a fusiform or globuliform proliferation.

Example: Female patient of 49 years with a tumour in the right frontotemporal region. Operated two years ago, died 18 months afterwards. Morphologically a glioblastoma multiforme with extensive astrocytic components, regions with numerous giant cells and other parts almost exclusively consisting of spindle cells. In addition there are many regressive changes, haemorrhages, necroses and much vascular and mesenchymal proliferation. The various cell structures of the original blastoma can all be recognized in the *in vitro* colonies, but there is no difference from culture to culture. The *in situ* regionally distributed different cytological elements are consistently found in every single culture, regardless of the demonstrated regions from which they originate.

We have to conclude from these facts that the human glioblastoma multiforme develops differently from the experimental mouse glioma after intracerebral application of cancerogens. Whereas the experimental brain tumour really seems to originate from a primary proliferation of heteromorphous elements adjacent to the implantation, the results of our tissue culture investigations strongly suggest a development of human spontaneous gliomas from a majority of homologous elements from a certain area of influence. Thus they would on the one hand correspond to the field theory of *Willis* and on the other be amenable to a cytological classification.

Statements with very far reaching implications, based on the results of experimental investigations which can be adequately assessed or proved only by those familiar with a highly specialized technique, demand not only a practical demonstration but a more detailed discussion of theoretical backgrounds than I can give you in the remaining few minutes. I will restrict myself to the problem of dedifferentiation which is of fundamental importance for the problem as to whether results obtained *in vitro* have any significance for *in situ* problems.

According to general opinion all tissues in culture must undergo increasing dedifferentiation. To what extent this nomicoplasia — as

Pomerat called it — develops, depends on the technique employed, and that it only seems to be valid for particle explantations with a high proliferation rate can be demonstrated by the cultivation of human meningioma tissue by different methods.

Proliferation and differentiation of tissues are inversely proportional. Anyone trying to determine the degree of differentiation in quickly growing cultures will always get completely negative results. In order to avoid these false negatives we have introduced in our experiments a biphasic mode of operation. A different composition of the nutrient fluid stops the cellular divisions and produces within the culture a stationary state, in which certain signs of cellular and histological differentiation not previously present, become demonstrable.

The changes in tissues *in vitro* may be divided into histological dedifferentiation, or better disorganisation, which can be extraordinarily pronounced in cultivated normal tissue, and true or cellular dedifferentiation, which rarely reaches a marked degree. Distinguishing between disorganisation and dedifferentiation — as first proposed by *Lumsden* — has proved very useful in the cultivation of cerebral neoplasms because we are dealing with a material already severely disorganized *in situ* which — apart from the glioblastoma multiforme — does not show any definite signs of cellular dedifferentiation. The rudimentary organisations of these blastomas, still existing *in situ* can easily be recognized within the cultures of the same tumours, provided these primary structures are not dependent on vascular formations which *in vitro* no longer exist.

Rudimentary organisations of this sort are the bundles of spongioblasts in cerebellar astrocytomas, the satellite formation in oligodendrogliomas, which is also to be found in normal foetal brain tissues, the fine reticular formation of cerebral astrocytoma, the rosette-like structures of ependymoma and the whorls in meningiomas. Only glioblastomas do not show any organisation. Their diagnosis *in vitro* is made by the high degree of cytoplasmic and nuclear anaplasia.

We conclude from these facts, that the rudimentary organisations of brain tumours are more deeply inherent at the cellular level than the functional organisations of normal tissues, which can rarely be reproduced *in vitro*.

Compared with the easily recognized disorganisation an increasing dedifferentiation of single cells is much more difficult to demonstrate. The relation between disorganisation and dedifferentiation being variable, a higher degree of disorganisation is no criterion for cellular dedifferentiation, by which we understand the constant loss of morphological and functional characteristics. The artificial environment of a culture, above all the change from three to two dimensions presents a strong challenge to the cells, the fatal effects of which they can only escape by an extensive adaption. A simplified cell formation *in vitro* therefore does not give very much information about the degree of dedifferentiation. Unfortunately the degree of preservation of functional powers despite morphological simplification of the cell cannot be exactly estimated because of the lack of proper stimuli. Thus the problem of dedifferentiation can only be studied in cells whose function is independent of external stimuli and results in a visible end product.

In the cultivation of human melanoblastomas and the pigmented epithelium of retina it can be demonstrated that these cells preserve their special ability in vitro for many months and that no important dedifferentiation takes place. Certainly these results cannot be directly applied to neuroectodermal neoplasms, but if — for example — the cells of a protoplasmic astrocytoma in vitro under increasing dilution of the nutrient fluid show an increasing transformation from spindle shaped cells to stellate astrocytes. I think we may conclude, that cellular dedifferentiation in primary cultures cannot play an important role.

Discussion

Dr. Zülch: We are faced again with a wealth of good observations that deserve long discussion. I think these observations can be discussed from three angles. One in relation to the genesis of tumours. The second may be academic or practical as you wish for I think Dr. Kersting's results will help us also to decide some of the open questions, for instance whether there is an astroblastoma and what the relation of astroblastoma to astrocytoma and to glioblastoma is and similar questions. And I am sure and everybody who knows his book will be sure that his contribution in the near future to these various open questions will be very valuable. And thirdly he has been — as the Anglosaxons say — playing already around in a similar way to Dr. Netsky in his experimental work and transplantations to study the cytostatic effects of various factors. Tissue cultures are very useful, as you said, for experimenting with various chemical drugs, with X-rays and all other sorts of radiation. I think we all thank you for your very good paper which is now open to discussion.

Dr. Calvo: It is extremely interesting that the form of the cell depends on the amount of fluid around it, — also the density of fluid, because it happens that in the grey matter we see the more stellate cells in astrocytomas. In the white matter which is more dense we find the fibrillary type including the pilocytic, piloid or spongioblast type, i. e. find it in the most dense parts of the brain, i. e. the optic tract and medulla.

Dr. Kersting: Well, to be precise the diluted fluid contains less nutrient media than the fluid which we use in the proliferation phase. I fear it has nothing to do with viscosity or anything that you might understand as density.

Dr. Rubinstein: What seems so valuable to me in this approach of tissue culture and the artificial production of tumours is that it throws so much more interesting a light upon the mode of growth ad spread of tumours than upon the question of semantics, and the influence of the environment upon the tumour cells is an important factor to our understanding. In the brain also you have cells which adapt their shape within structures and one is familiar of course with gliomas which have quite a different structure whether they are primary tumours or secondary metastases.

Dr. Zülch: Thank you, Dr. Rubinstein. Will you answer, Dr. Kersting?

Dr. Kersting: What I am saying is that quite a lot of people concerned with tissue culture use now the word nomikoplasia, a law abiding differentiation which in fact is almost 90% dependent on what you do, on what technique you use. And before you have used several techniques, it is quite impossible for you to know how things will develop. They develop differently on every occasion, and what I wanted to emphasize are the fundamental differences between a quick growing and a slow growing transplant or culture. So if Dr. Netsky said that if you do those very quick series of transplantations then you get spongio-blastomas and if you don't make quick transplantations you get astrocytomas, that is only a result of the rapidity of growth and nothing else. And that is, I think, the point, where the experiments with the cancerogenous introduction of brain tumour and tissue culture become crucial.

Dr. Netsky: To me it is most interesting that the results you presented are in agreement with so much of what I presented and I think they are mutually interchangeable. The tumour cells are the victims of their environment. It may be that some of the differences we have seen, as Dr. Rubinstein said, are really dependent on environment, the rate at which the cells are growing, the phase in which they are growing, and so on. Many of these differences may well be resolved, when we can understand or define the conditions of growth in human tumours as well as in experimental tumours.

Dr. Calvo: I would like to ask Dr. Kersting if the cells that grow in astrocytic form and then have been in a diluted medium grow slower than the spindle cells.

Dr. Kersting: They don't grow at all. That is a stationary state. They do not divide any more.

Dr. Calvo: So they have all the differentiation of structure of an astrocyte.

Dr. Kersting: That's what I mean.

Dr. Liss: I would like to ask you if I may say that it was not only a beautiful scientific presentation but also an aesthetic pleasure to see the growing cells. It is the fate of the histologist to kill the cells before he can determine how they would look in life and we should not forget in our enthusiasm that there are several points about which we have to be very cautious in evaluating tissue cultures. Dr. Kersting is, I think, using this caution to a great extent, but as far as the diagnostic value of tissue culture is concerned we have been able to observe that if we use a maintenance culture from the beginning and watch the behavior of the migrating cells, these cells have many typical characteristics peculiar to the type of tumour, so that in many cases it has been a very valuable help, mainly in cases where there was a differential diagnostic point, for example especially if we are dealing with a uniform type of mixed tumour — and some-how we believe that in these cases the actual blastomatous cell grows much more vigorously in the maintenance culture from the beginning and that it is the one which migrates first and dominates the entire picture of the culture.

Dr. Kersting: I would support what Dr. Liss said if he means the mixed tumour or tumour in which there are different cell types. Some may be more vigorous and others less, but this sort of approach may lead to pit falls and I think we have shown this with the cerebellar astrocytoma. If you take a cerebellar astrocytoma and make it grow then it grows like a spongioblastoma and if you bring it into a stationary state it will not develop into stellate astrocytes at all, it remains a spongioblastoma. But if you from the beginning only work with higher dilutions of nutrient fluid there will migrate a few stellate astrocytes and that is probably why Dr. Dorothy Russell years ago said that there is no difference between the cerebellar astrocytoma and the cerebral astrocytoma. I can't give you the reason for it now, but there is a definite difference between cerebellar astrocytoma and cerebral astrocytoma that is, if you start with a proliferation phase; during the stationary phase the cerebral astrocytoma shows these stellate astrocytes, the cerebellar astrocytoma does not.

Dr. Rubinstein: Your observations, Dr. Kersting, are extremely interesting. In the thirties there were different technical methods and this may account for the differences in results. Your suggestion about these presumably preexisting astrocytes is an interesting one, but the Bergmann glia is normally piloid anywhere, and is in fact a mature glial cell.

Dr. Zülch: Any other comments? Then I thank you again and I call upon Dr. Woolf.

5. Electron Microscopy

Remarks on the Electronmicroscopical Appearances of Brain Tumours

By

A. L. Woolf

When I first heard that this Symposium was going to take place I was working and in fact we had been working for some time on the electronmicroscopy of the intramuscular nerve endings and on cutaneous nerves taken at biopsy. I told Dr. *Zülch* that I was of course as a neuropathologist extremely interest in cerebral tumours and as an expression of gratitude for the chance to come and hear what people said during the Symposium, I would carry out electronmicroscopy on some cerebral tumours for him. Now, I am sure you realize how very difficult it is to switch from the tissue that you are most interested in to another and just as we were starting to collect some cerebral tumour material to study with the electronmicroscope, we ran into some domestic difficulties in the laboratory so I am only able to show you our first preparations, but rather than back out of my commitment and leave the Symposium without reference being made to electronmicroscopy and its potential value for you, I thought the best thing to do would be to make a survey of the work which has been done by other electronmicrocopists on cerebral tumours so you could see the value of the method. When I went through the literature I found that the task was much easier than I had anticipated because on the one hand electronmicroscopic technique has developed so rapidly that the one or two early attempts at carrying out these studies did not really give us anything of interest and secondly even in recent years as far as published work is concerned almost no one has occupied himself with this matter. And in fact what I am going to do apart from passing round photographs of my own preparations which are easier for you to see than when they are just flashed on the screen, is to take you through the only comprehensive study in the literature on this subject. Now I will pass round the photographs so you have them with you while I am talking. The two pictures here are from normal mouse brain, actually this one here shows a large nerve cell in the middle which is not of great interest, but in the corner here is the network of structures that one has to try and unravel in doing electronmicroscopy of normal and pathological brains. And here is a high magnification of an area which is made up of glial processes. These are normal ones. The other two photographs are both taken from an astrocytoma, a very fibre forming type of astrocytoma from the cerebral hemisphere of a young child, and I want you to notice particularly the appearance of the fibre processes of fibrillary astrocytes in tumours, which I think is of some interest and may be helpful in diagnosis to supplement staining methods which are perhaps not of absolutely proven specificity for fibres. What is perhaps more important is the appearance in the cytoplasm of a tumour astrocyte of very much larger numbers of mitochondria than you normally find and also that the mitochondria appear to be either of two types or in two phases. Some of them are dark and some are lighter, and it may well be that this type of tumour will give us some insight into what makes the cell malignant or what makes a cell neoplastic. The only comprehensive work on this subject is in "Neurology" (1960) by *Sarah Luse* * and it will be interesting if I just go over her preparations. Now what she shows first is an appearance very similar to that shown on the photograph passed round. This is a normal protoplasmic astrocyte. You may feel that with the electronmicroscope you are not seeing so much more than what you can see with standard methods. There are a few things that you notice. Here of course you see the nucleus with a little chromatin in it and what she stresses are these little processes which are the processes of the cytoplasm of the astrocyte. Now of course in this way electronmicroscopy I think almost gives us less to see than with light microscope methods because of course the sections are so thin, you can't see the processes as a whole. Now down below here is a possibly fibrous astrocyte and its fibrous nature is established beyond doubt by the appearance of the astrocytic fibres. Now to prove it — and I think it does prove it, — she shows a section here from the brain of an animal which has had a glial scar produced by injection of aluminia gel. You see that there are a great many of the structures and I think it is quite acceptable that this is the appearance of astrocytic fibres and you will remember that they were very prominent in the photograph I passed round which of course was a very fibrillary astrocytoma, which all adds to the probability of their being astrocytic fibres. And in the first tumour she shows you see the type of astrocyte and you probably agree that it shows very much more of the characteristic features of these

---

* See: *Luse, S. A.,* Neurology, Minneapolis, *10* (1960), 88.

processes than you would see with the light microscope. I think it is interesting to see what a "gemästete" astrocyte cell looks like and here is one. You can't again say much about the processes which are small but it is interesting to see this granular material which is responsible for the hyaline appearance of the cells in comparison with the light microscope view. This is the first of the structures which are as yet unidentifiable, again in an astrocytoma, and so far, we don't know what their nature is but Dr. Luse thinks it might be the beginning of the microcystic changes which are common in these tumours. Here is a cell from a glioblastoma and you see as of course you would see with the ordinary microscope the irregularly shaped nucleus, but what she thinks is interesting and I don't know if it should have surprised one, is the presence of fibrils within the processes. She rather stresses this as being particularly interesting and as showing that a glioblastoma cell is related to astrocyte cells, but you may think that because the cell is present in a glioblastoma it is not necessarily a tumour cell. In this next photograph, the electron-microscope appearance of this type of nucleus is just as you would expect, but what I do think is interesting is the very large number of mitochondria which you can find as I have shown not only in a glioblastoma but also in an astrocytoma cell and I think that there should be some attempt to correlate this finding with studies by cell fractionation and enzyme studies of the activity of the mitochondria.

I expect you would be interested to see what the oligodendroglia look like. As you might have expected they have a remarkably clear cytoplasm. This is a normal one here and that clear appearance is also present in this blastomatous oligodendrocyte. Dr. Luse makes no comments on these nuclei, I can't explain why there are so many nuclei in a cell from a tumour which she shows in another place with a light microscope as having only one nucleus in each cell, but that is the appearance of the oligodendroglioma cell. Now these are oligodendroglioma cells and these are not nuclei, they are very large mitochondria and this is a nucleolus from an oligodendroglioma cell which I don't think is so interesting; and there are again large numbers of mitochondria. I think the mitochondria are very interesting because we don't see them in light microscopy and they have surely something very important to do with the rate of growth.

This is a choroid plexus papilloma, but the appearance of the cells, according to Dr. Luse, is very similar to that of ependymoma cells and the characteristic features are microvilli and cilia as you see within the cytoplasm and the fact that the cytoplasm is so electron dense is according to Dr. Luse due to a lot of ribonucleo-protein. This might be useful, I think, in diagnosis.

This diapositive is from an ependymoma. It shows the cilia very well and the type of nucleus which she says is particularly characteristic of this tumour. The feature which Dr. Luse says is particularly characteristic about the meningioma shown here is the interdigitating of the cytoplasmic processes of the tumour cells. It is much closer interdigitation than in the astrocytomas and she says probably it is responsible for the whorled appearance. This is a neurofibroma, there is a myelin sheath with this axon and these are collagen fibres. She does not show reticulin fibres, but the possibility of distinction between reticulin fibres and glial fibres is very important and should be valuable. This is a neurilemmoma, where again you get a certain amount of interdigitation of the processes but not as marked as in a meningioma. I am afraid that is really all I can say, all that there is to say. I hope I have indicated that the field is a profitable one and I am sure at the moment quite a number of different centres have already accumulated some useful preparations.

Discussion

Dr. Zülch: Thank you very much, Dr. Woolf, for your bird's eye view and report on this very important line of research which is however just developing and as you frankly admitted there is not too much that can be said at the moment. But I think in the long run there will be a wealth of information available from this method, for instance one question has always interested me whether the so called fibres in neurinoma are actually reticulin fibres or whether they are only a condensation of the Schwann cell sheath. This might easily be decided on the basis of electronmicroscopic observations. So I see very many problems which one ought to tackle and may be able to solve by this method. I wonder if anybody wants to comment on this. Dr. Wechsler has some experience in normal brains.

Dr. Wechsler: I would like to refer to experiments I made with Dr. Hager in Munich. My present interest is particularly in peripheral nerves and muscles, not the central nervous system and I think the task of determining for instance whether glial cells are derived from tumours or are reactive is a very difficult one. As far as I know from the pictures of Hager, who has done a great deal of work on brain trauma, brain inflammation and virus inflammation where there also occur a lot of reactive processes and also I know the publications of Sarah Luse, and she again emphazises the difficulty in distinguishing between reactive and neoplastic astrocytes. I think the future will show if electronmicroscopy will bring you information on these problems. I am sure there are some questions existing which are much easier to solve, for instance in peripheral nerve it is easy to distinguish between Schwann cells and derivates from the mesenchyme and I would like to say let us wait and see.

Dr. Rubinstein: There is one aspect in the electronmicroscopy of tumours which is already giving us a fascinating glimps as to its possibilities. I refer to Sarah Luse's finding of these large abnormal mitochondria in the oligodendrogliomas. We can correlate this observation with the work done in 1939 by Victor and Wolf in New York and later on by Elliott in Montreal regarding the respiratory capacity of human brain tumours. The astrocytomas and glioblastomas had a respiratory quotient much lower than normal, the oligodendrogliomas a much higher respiratory quotient. This is a problem where electronmicroscopy may give us the greatest amount of information.

Dr. Wechsler: A short remark on the accumulation of mitochondria. For instance we have studied in Munich the process of regeneration in neurons and if you look at the tip of regenerating neurons, the so called growing cone, you can observe that there is an axoplasm very rich in mitochondria and very rich in so called endoplasmic reticulum and vesicles. All these three components are found in normal axons too but to a much lesser degree. We also know this from Gasser's electronmicroscopic studies of embryonic cells and differentiating cells i. e. growing cells and the process of growing is naturaly correlated with an increase in mitochondria and it is very difficult to accept that this belongs to what in biochemical terms is a process of metabolism belonging specifically to blastoma cells. It is more a process of growing in blastoma cells and one should emphazise that electronmicroscopy is a morphological method and all conclusions made on morphological observation should be restricted to this aspect of the problem.

Dr. Zülch: Thank you for your critical remarks. There was one thing that struck me, the gemistocytic astrocyte was full of mitochondria, wasn't that so?

Dr. Woolf: Not a great number, there were some other structures, I have forgotten the word, Dr. Luse used.

Dr. Zülch: Any other questions? We now have Dr. Müller's paper on the histochemical examination of brain tumours.

Remarks on the Histochemistry of Brain Tumours

By

W. Müller*

With 3 Figures

While routine staining techniques are suitable for demonstrating the distribution of substrate, histochemical methods should help to clarify, through analysis of the basic components, structural relationships particularly in cases where the problem of metabolic dynamics is in the foreground. A large number of biochemical analyses have been applied in adapted form to histological sections. Particularly in the last decade new histochemical techniques have been developed and are already used as a routine. During the 4th Neuropathology Congress at Munich in 1961 a series of papers dealt with the problems of histochemistry of brain tumours.

The studies frequently showed contradictory results. The cause for this lies in the different methods used by various workers. Without referring in detail to the principles underlying the methods used in histochemical work it will be mentioned that different methods require special fixation of the tissue, as has been known for a long time in regard to the demonstration of glycogen. The method of native-slides, the preparation of the material with the cryostat, or the freezing drying-method are not valid for all histochemical investigations.

The tissue by its very nature contains another factor which introduces difficulties in the use of histochemical methods for brain tumours or brain tissue.

The majority of observations especially in enzyme histochemistry have been made on kidney or liver. In applying the methods to brain tissue some modifications have, of course, been made, but without changing the principles. As one cannot expect any far reaching contribution to the problem of classification from histochemistry, I wish to demonstrate a few examples which bear little direct relationship to the spirit of this symposium.

---

* *Müller, W.*, and *H. Nasu*, Enzymhistochemische Untersuchungen an Gliomen. Die Naturwissensch. *49* (1962), 496—497.

We have often found in the neurinomas a gold-brown, granular pigment, which has been recognized as haematogenous pigment because of the positive reaction for iron. In our studies we concluded that it was a lipopigment and not a blood pigment.

Among the differential reactions Fig. 1 shows the positive Fontana reaction, which demonstrates the reductive power of this pigment.

This statement naturally leads to the next question of the origin of the pigment in the neurinomas. Studies on the so-called lipid neurinoma, i. e. the Type B of *Antoni,* by our collaborator

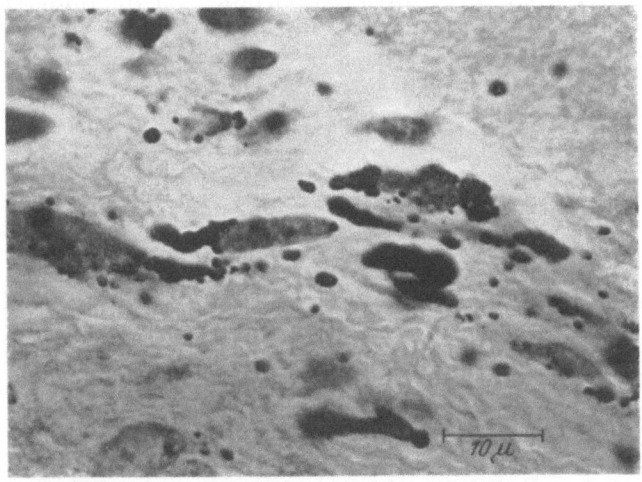

Fig. 1. Fontana's reaction on the pigment in the cells of a neurinoma.

Dr. *Hegedus* showed the lipid substances to be a complex mixture, in which the same substances can be found as in the degeneration of myelin. The connection between this observation and the lipid nature of the pigment is obvious (Fig. 2).

Other parallels were shown by comparison between the tissue of neurinoma and myelinated nerve fibres, with which the cells of Schwann are associated. The fibres in the neurinoma are still discussed frequently. From their histochemical behaviour their nature must be mesodermal. Other supplementary studies on this tumour suggest the following concept of the neurinoma: primarily the tumour is built up of Schwann cells, in which we find a few fibrocytes, surrounding the parenchymatous cells (i. e. the Schwann cells) with a dense fibre-network.

Because of their biological potentialities the Schwann cells yield
lipid substances, which are necessary to the myelin sheaths of
normal nerve fibres.

As we definitely know from electron-microscopic studies, when
a myelin sheath is formed in the presence of an axon, the amount
of the lipids and prelipids grows and leads finally to the type B
neurinoma, in which in the same tissue degeneration of lipids
occurs.

Whether the mesodermal cells are responsible for the transport
or the cells of Schwann themselves wander in an amoeboid manner
to the vessel (which may be possible according to the studies of
Weiss and *Wang*) this is of no importance for the understanding of

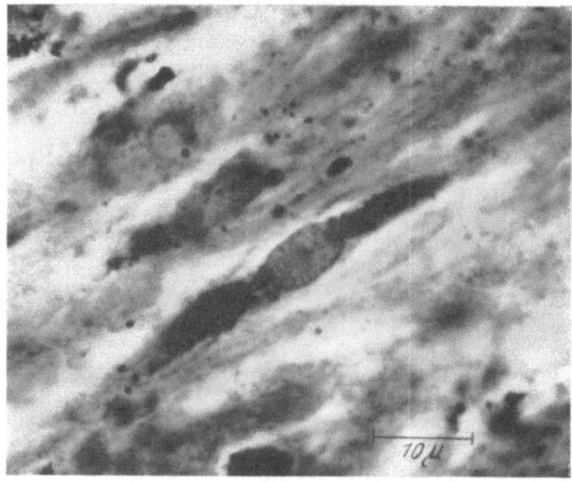

Fig. 2. Sudan-black colouration of granular material in the cyptoplasm on bcth sides of thc
nucleus. Compare with Fig. 1.

the biology of the neurinoma. Because the mesodermal elements in
the tumour grow, it gives the picture of a fibromatous tumour.
Histochemical studies also make a contribution to this hypothesis.

The accepted picture of type A and B is seen in the same tumour,
because the dynamics of the tumour behave differently in different
parts at the same time, reflecting only the biological situation at a
particular moment. Surveying the series of studies, concerned with
the pigment, this example shows the real problem for histochemical
methods.

Earlier histological staining and endocrinological studies have
shown us, that the present classification of the tumours of the pituitary are not in accordance with the clinical picture. We are forced

by our studies to grade many adenomas as chromophobe when their cytology shows signs of secretory activity. Among the signs of cell-activity is, in particular, richness of cytoplasmic RNA.

Of course, the difference can only be made evident by special fixation and staining with Gallocyanin-Chrome-Alum (Fig. 3). The difference is even more evident after fluorochromating with acridin-orange.

Schümmelfeder studied intensively the physicochemical correlations and the specifity of the method for nucleic acids, in a series

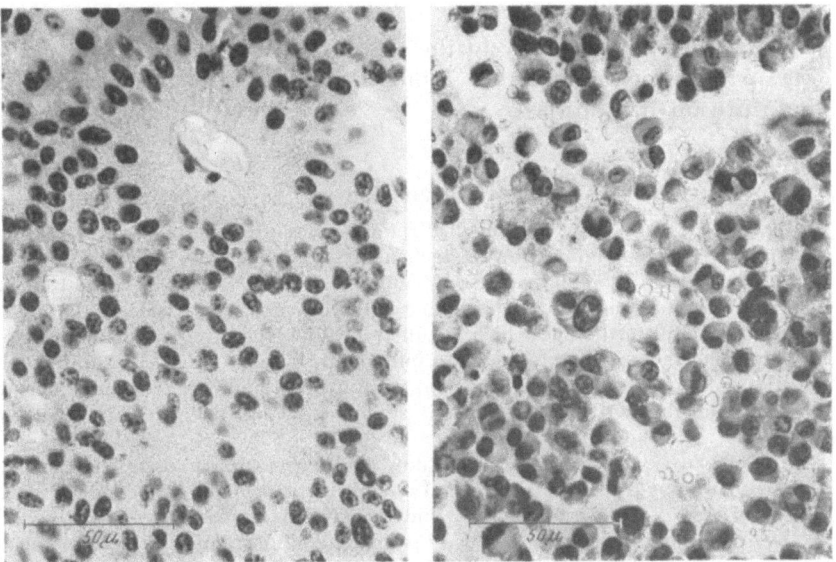

Fig. 3. Gallocyanin-Chrome-Alum staining for the detection of RNA in pituitary adenomas. Left: chromophobe adenoma. Right: mixed type adenoma. In the latter the high degree of cytoplasmic RNA is obvious.

of special studies on other material. I only mention the use of ribo-nuclease to ensure the results. I would now like to draw attention to other studies, which don't help to solve the problem of classi-fication, but give some clues as to the origin of the tumour tissue.

So for example, our former coworker Dr. *Fotakis* described "Cell inclusions" (Zelleinschlüsse) in gangliocytomas, which look like neurosecreting material on staining and histochemically. As we know from other studies that neurosecreting nuclei are phylo-genetically old, it seems to us a not unjustified hypothesis that one part of gangliocytomas is not only an ontogenetic dysformation, but may also be a phylogenetic atavism.

6*

The enzyme histochemistry work of our coworker Dr. *Nasu* proves correlations between the ferment content of the embryonal tissue on the one hand and medulloblastoma and ependymoma on the other. These results were completed by the fact that the ependymoma gives a similar positive reaction for cholinesterase, to that shown by the ependyma of mammalian and human embryos. The ependyma of adult man and animal is always negative. The studies of Dr. *Viale* completed these results with further details, but their discussion would be too detailed for this contribution.

A large number of these histochemical results are identical with the biochemical reports.

This report refers only to the studies which were carried out at our institute, and for further details I would like to refer you to the literature on this subject.

Discussion

Dr. Zülch: Thank you very much, Dr. Müller, for giving us so many examples in which you have shown how histochemistry can help in either classification of a tumour or in the solution of academic questions or even throw light on the biology of the tumours. In my discussion with you yesterday I learned that histochemistry is still in the age which is called in philosophy: phenomenology. They just describe facts and only begin to understand what it means. I think it was most stimulating to hear you and I am waiting for comments from the audience on this contribution of Dr. Müller. Has anyone experience in histochemistry? Or would anyone like to comment?

Dr. Wechsler: I would like to know if there are any differences in the behavior of dehydrogenases in normal oligodendrocytes and oligodendrogliomas.

Dr. Müller: We have an increase but the differences are not marked.

Dr. Wechsler: I ask this because in the earlier discussion on electronmicroscopy it was emphazised that according to Dr. Luse there is a marked increase of mitochondria in the oligodendroglia of the oligodendroglioma. There is a good deal of evidence that there is a very strong correlation between the increase of mitochondria seen in electronmicroscopy and studies with histochemical methods. Therefore it is interesting to hear that Dr. Müller has now observed significant differences in normal and neoplastic oligodendrocytes.

Dr. Zülch: Is there anybody else who wants to comment on this? Thank you very much and I am now calling on Dr. Calvo.

7. Metallic Impregnation

Observations on the Metallic Impregnations of Brain Tumours

By

W. Calvo*

With 5 Figures

The metallic impregnations, largely developed by the Spanish school, have greatly increased our knowledge of the morphology of the tumours of nervous tissue. Whenever we wish to trace the cell type from which a neoplasm originates we have to use a method endowed with a maximum of specificity. This specificity is found in some of the methods in which the essential feature is the selective impregnation of the cells by a heavy metal. A variety of solutions of gold and silver participate in the "modus operandi" of the methods described by *Cajal, Hortega, Achúcarro* and others during the first quarter of this century. The reduced silver nitrate of *Cajal* for the demonstration of neurofibrils, the sublimate gold chloride of *Cajal* for astroglia, the tannin silver of *Achúcarro* for reticulin and the silver carbonate of *Hortega* for the demonstration of oligodendroglia and microglia are the fundamental metallic impregnations for the characterization of the different elements of the nervous tissue and they are, therefore, the methods most able to give us a clue as to the classification of a neoplasm on a morphological basis. It is somewhat more difficult to master these techniques than to stain with haematoxylin-eosin, but it is my experience that any well trained technician can produce good preparations after a few days practice.

The reasons underlying the reluctance of most laboratories of neuropathology to stain neoplasms of nervous tissue routinely with metallic impregnations extend beyond the lack of good laboratory technicians. More important is the special attention that must be given to each section requiring much time for its completion and the special requirements for fixation of the tissue. On many occasions we have to prepare tissues fixed in conditions far from ideal or already embedded in paraffin or celloidin (these are the main

* *Calvo, W.,* Tumores Encefalomedulares. Arch. españ. morfol. 1954.

obstacles to good impregnation); in addition, there is, in many cases, insufficient material for fixing the tissue in two fixatives: formalin and formol-bromide as is required ideally. Taking these facts into consideration we must compromise and try to get the best results possible in every case of the routine work of the laboratory, keeping the original methods as given by the old masters for special research work.

It is true that haematoxylin-eosin gives enough information in most cases to permit a diagnosis, but whenever we wish to discuss a case, classify an unusual sample, or work on taxonomy, we have to go back to the more specific methods.

The minimum requirements for routine work in a laboratory of neuropathology should be, in our opinion, one section stained with *Mallory's* phosphotungstic acid-haematoxylin and one section stained with a metallic impregnation demonstrating collagen and reticulin fibers without destroying the cells. If the tissue is embedded in paraffin or celloidin *Wilder's* method for reticulin gives the best results even in very old material. The connective tissue is shown very distinctly and the relations between cells and fibres can easily be studied if phosphotungstic acid is used instead of permanganate as sensitizer in the first step. The relation between cells and connective tissue fibres is very important for the diagnosis of sarcomas. The cytoplasm of the cells can be shown much better if the section is counterstained with amido-black in acid solution — we have demonstrated the excellence of this dye as a cytoplasmic stain. The background is clean, and it is easy to avoid precipitates. The nuclei of the cells are visible. This enables a general survey to be made of the main elements of the connective tissue and the neoplastic cells. A third slide may be necessary in order to demonstrate Nissl substance or neurofibrils. A good stain for the neurons in material embedded in celloidin or paraffin is the method of *Schultze-Gross*.

Material embedded in paraffin is inadequate for a good demonstration of the oligodendroglia and microglia, but where no fresh tissue is available acceptable results may be contained with the silver tungstate of *Grino* or with a modification of *Penfield* to *Hortega's* method. This modification gave acceptable impregnations in the hands of Dr. *Meller* * even in old material fixed in formalin and embedded in paraffin. The cytoplasm and processes of the

---

* See: *Meller, K.*, Modifikation der Silberimprägnation zur Darstellung der Zellen des Oligodendroglioms im Paraffinmaterial. Acta neuropath. 2 (1963), 497—500.

oligodendroglia appear black against a greyish background. The nuclei are unstained.

In more favourable cases where non-embedded formalin fixed and formol-bromide fixed tissue is available, the formalin fixed tissue may be used for the demonstration of ganglion cells and the tissue fixed in formol-bromide for impregnation of glia. Where only one fixative may be chosen, we recommend formol-bromide for neoplasms of the nervous tissue. The fixation can be corrected later if necessary, if it is desired to stain the neurofibrils. Many good methods are available for the demonstration of neurofibrils in frozen sections: *Bielschowsky, Gross* or double impregnation of *Hortega* give consistent results.

Cajal described a silver oxide method that is not well known but is, in our opinion, very important for the study of neoplasms of the nervous system, because with this method the astrocytes and connective tissue are both beautifully impregnated. It is almost as good as the gold sublimate chloride for astrocytes and better than many special stains for the demonstration of the reticulin. It tolerates a much longer period of fixation than the gold sublimate and stains cells of a more immature type — therefore it constitutes an ideal method for the study of tumours of nervous tissue. With the silver oxide of *Cajal* the fibrillary astrocytes and the connective tissue can easily be demonstrated many years after fixation in formol-bromide. The protoplasmic astrocytes and the most undifferentiated cytoplasm of some neoplastic cells lose their argentophilia after a few months of fixation. The cytoplasm of normal oligodendrocytes is not impregnated. The nuclei of all the cells can be stained after many years of fixation. The *Rosenthal* fibers are beautifully impregnated. In the ependymal series the rapidly growing neoplasms have cells with faintly stained cytoplasmic processes but in more mature ependymal elements the relation of the vascular feet with the blood vessels is very well demonstrated. With this method alone diagnosis of most of the tumours of the nervous tissue with an accurate analysis of their most important histological features is possible. A combination of silver oxide for one slide and cresyl violet for another is strongly recommended.

For the selective demonstration of oligodendrocytes it is necessary to impregnate sections with *Hortega's* silver carbonate but if the tissue has been fixed for a long time in formalin-bromide or initially fixed in formalin it is necessary to apply the modification of *Penfield. Hortega's* silver carbonate also demonstrates the microglia simply by varying the manner of reduction of the sections. *Hortega's* silver carbonate is not absolutely specific for the oligodendroglia. Some astrocytes around the arterioles and precapillaries of the cortex are also stained, but the intimate relations of these cells with the blood vessels and the morphological characteristics of the astrocytes makes it easy to recognize both of them. The neurons are faintly stained and only the body but not the fibres can be seen. The glioblasts and most of the neoplastic cells of other groups are very lightly impregnated, while the oligodendrocytes show a dense black cytoplasm around a rounded unstained nucleus. Not all the neoplastic oligodendrocytes are impregnated. Some of them show only a narrow ring of cytoplasm or appear as "naked" nuclei. This may be due to absence of argentophilia of some imma- ture cells or to the fact that many oligodendrocytes show a definite polarization of the cytoplasm that may lay across the section so that the nucleus and the cytoplasm can be in two different sections. The oligodendrocytes can be recognized by the clear rounded nucleus and heavily stained cytoplasm. Sometimes the cytoplasm is abun- dant and angular with a few thin expansions in which corkscrew formations can be distinguished and a few branches, but never pro- ducing vascular feet. Some other neoplastic oligodendrocytes have very few and short expansions and a narrow ring of cytoplasm.

Hortega's silver carbonate for astrocytes gives a very good im- pregnation of the astroglia but the silver oxide of Cajal is just as good for the demonstration of the astroglia, and has the advantage of a much better impregnation of the connective tissue.

The sublimate gold chloride of Cajal is the most specific of the metallic methods for the demonstration of astroglia, because only astrocytes, astroblasts and blood vessels can be impregnated. The reactive astrocytes are the most heavily stained, to a less extent the normal astrocytes and less than the normal the neoplastic astro- cytes. The oligodendrocytes and microglia show only their nuclei. The soma of the neurons appears very pale, but their expansions cannot be seen. The limitations of the sublimate gold chloride with respect to the short time of fixation required in formalin-bromide are greatly reduced by Hortega's modification which permits the use of material fixed for longer periods.

Now I would like to show a few slides stained with metallic impregnations. The first is a sarcoma with wide blood vessels and formation of a very dense mesh of reticulin. In the second we can see a much denser reticulin mesh in another sarcoma; the cells lie in small boxes produced by the mesh-work of the reticulin (Fig. 1). The third is a section with a few oligodendrocytes. There is a clear space in which the nucleus lies with a few very short expansions. Some cells have two nuclei and longer expansions (Fig. 2). This is

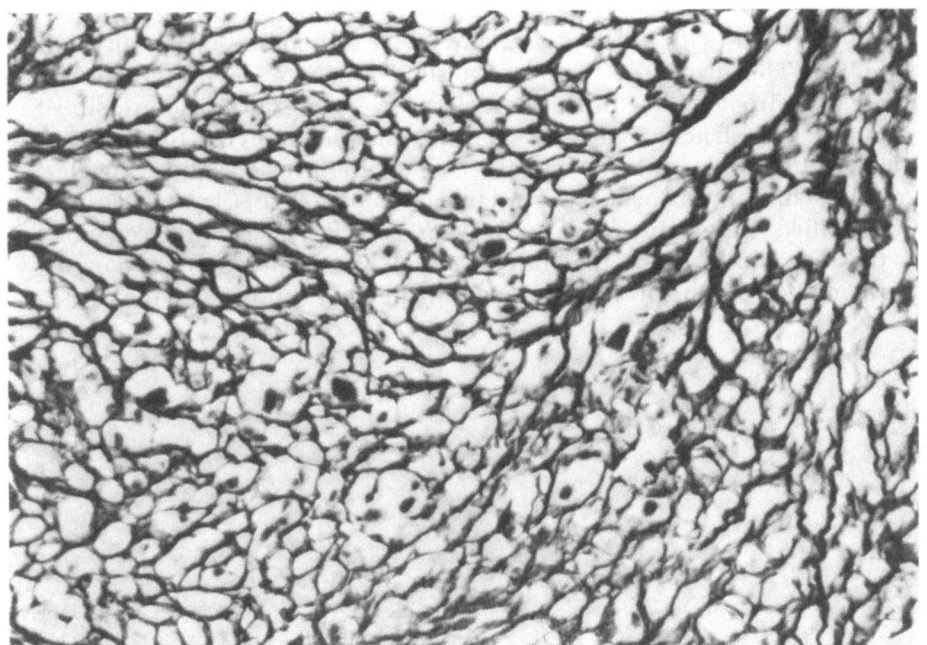

Fig. 1. Sarcoma of right occipital lobe showing a dense mesh-work of reticulin surrounding each cell. Oc. 10 ×; Ob. 25 ×. *Wilder's* method, paraffin section. formalin fixed material.

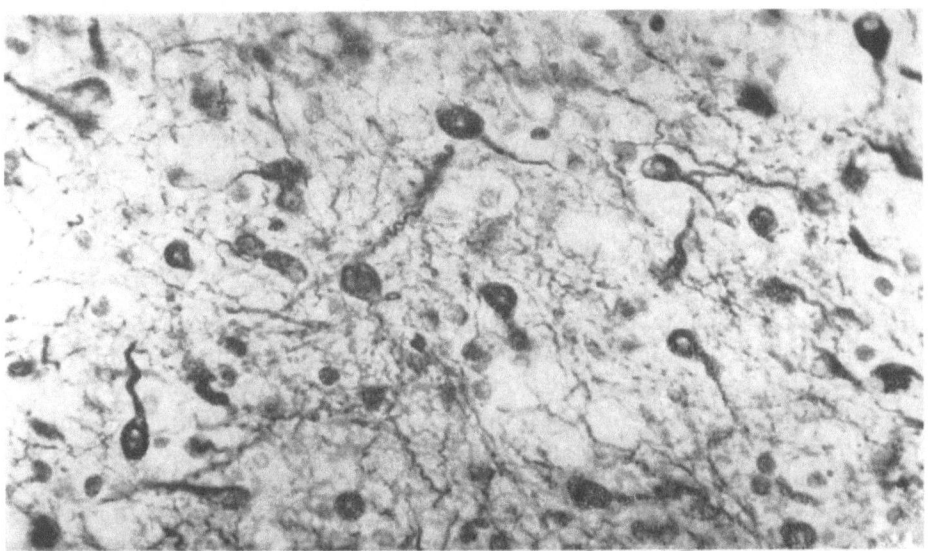

Fig. 2. Oligodendrocytoma of the frontal lobes. Oligodendrocytes with clear nuclei, very few expansions and some corkscrew formation. Oc. 10 ×; Ob. 20 ×. *Hortega's* silver carbonate, frozen section, formalin-bromide fixed material.

another cell with two nuclei, and here is another one with two nuclei. The neoplasm in the next slide is a more densely cellular oligodendrocytoma and this cell shows a corkscrew structure similar to the structure that in normal oligodendrocytes follows the nerve fibres. In contrast with the cells of the previous slide, the elements of the next slide are attached to blood vessels and can be classified as astrocytes. As you can see, it is easy to recognize the many expansions that have been clearly impregnated. Some of them show gliofibrils and throughout the field can be seen the dense

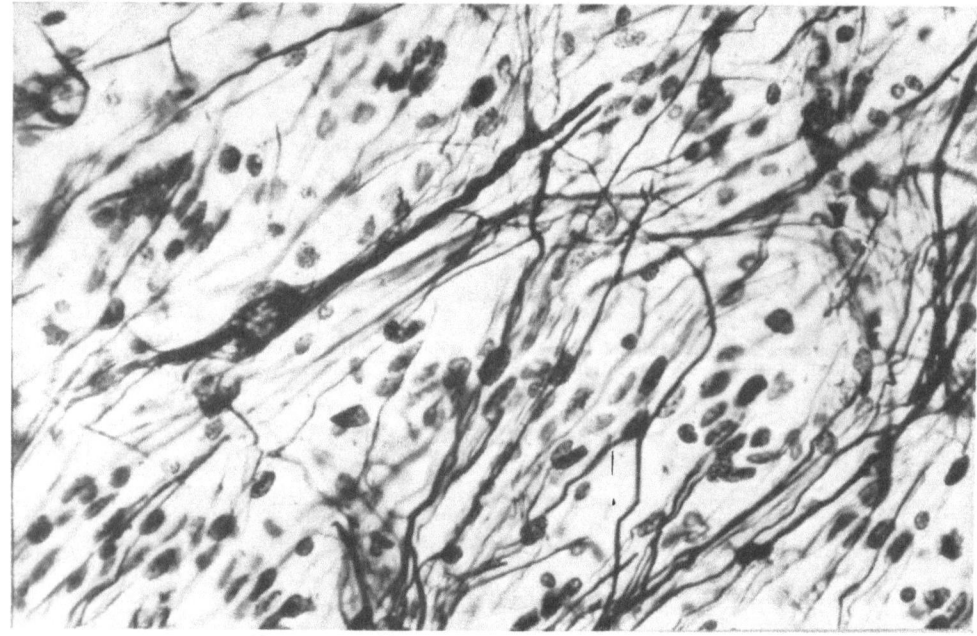

Fig. 3. Astrocytoma of cerebellum. The cells are bipolar and show gliofibrils. Oc. 10 ×; Ob. 20 ×. *Cajal's* silver oxide, formalin-bromide fixed material, frozen section.

plexiform organization of these cells with their expansions intermixed with one another. In the next slide the reticulin was impregnated by *Wilder's* method. Reticulin is present only on the wall of the blood vessels and no other reticulin could be found in this tumour, which was classified as a glioblastoma. Here a few cells send sucker feet to the blood vessels and a few giant cells are more distant but still attached to the wall of the blood vessels. In the next slide the reticulin in an ependymoma shows this dense mesh-work of fibres on the wall of the blood vessels. There is a clear space between the blood vessel and the nuclei. This space is occupied by the thin glial expansions that attach the cell to the wall of the blood vessel which is more clearly shown here. The most interesting feature of the ependymoma in the next slide is that it shows a surface of glial epithelium together with these tubes and vesicles of neuro-epithelium. But it also shows these fibres, *Rosenthal* fibres, that are clearly related to the glial epithelium. So these cells have two poles, one of the epithelial type and the other of glial type. We consider these expansions as glial because they are attached to the wall of

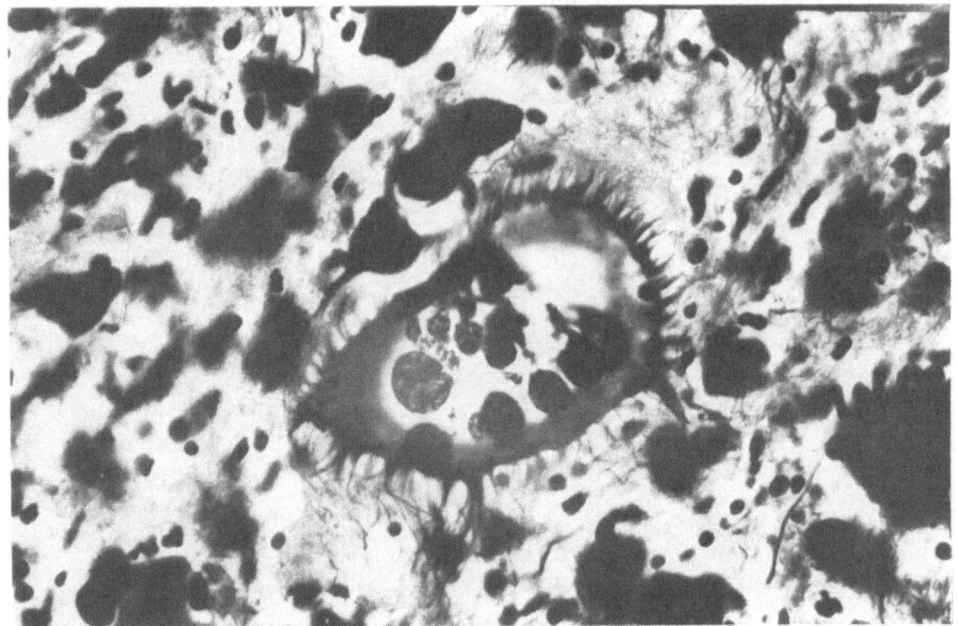

Fig. 4. Glioblastoma of frontal lobe. Giant multinucleated cell with numerous thin spike-like projections of cytoplasm and budding of the nuclei. Oc. 10 ×; Ob. 20 ×. *Cajal's* silver oxide, formalin-bromide fixation, frozen section.

the blood vessel. The absence of this glial expansion, with predominance of the epithelial architecture produces an ependymoma of the so called cellular type. But if these cells lose contact with the surface of the ependyma, the glial architecture predominates and the neoplasm is then the glial type of ependymoma. We may find also a mixture of both types. In the next slide, there is a higher magnification that shows in clearer detail these fibres going to the blood vessels and the neuroepithelium forming this surface. The next slide shows an example of an astrocytoma of the cerebellum in which we can see the glial fibres clearly stained and we can also see polar

cells or cells that could be considered as astroblasts because there
is a long expansion on this side of the cell and a few short expansions on the opposite side resembling those of the astroblasts
(Fig. 3). The next slide shows cells of the same type that may be
compared with astroblasts. Another field of the same tumour shows
elongated fusiform cells and other cells that resemble astroblasts.
The next slide shows a glioblastoma. The cells in the vicinity of the
blood vessel are very difficult to stain because their expansions are
granular. But there is some connection of some of the expansions
to the blood vessel wall. The next case shows another field of glio-

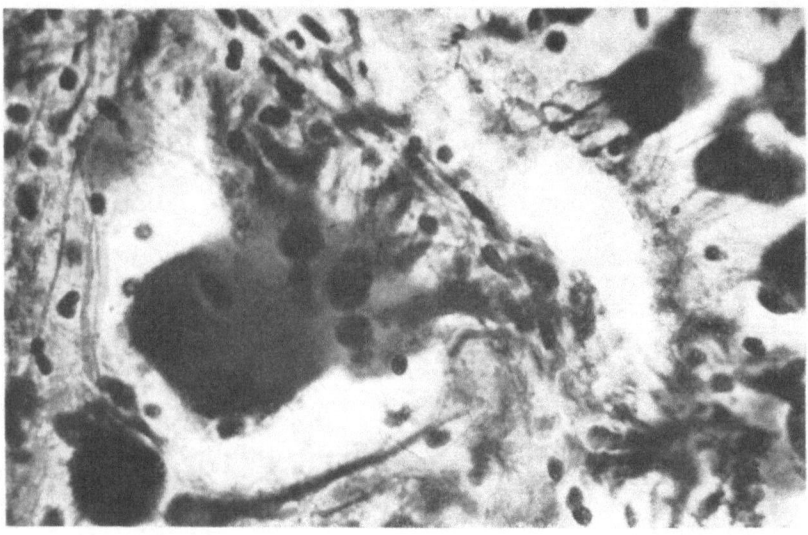

Fig. 5. Glioblastcma of frontal lobe. Giant multinucleated cell attached to a blood vessel by
numerous short processes. Oc. 10 ×; Ob. 20 ×. *Cajal's* silver oxide, formalin-bromide fixation,
frozen section.

blastoma in which you see many different types of cells with a
most unusual appearance. For example this one has a bulky cytoplasm with a few short expansions and this other one is difficult to
compare with any normal element. In the next slide we see a monster
cell from a glioblastoma and the interesting feature of this cell is
the very short and thin expansions which are very difficult to stain
by other methods (Fig. 4). It has to be a very selective or a very
special technique for showing these very faint thin and short expansions — otherwise the cell looks like a round balloon with several
enormous nuclei. You can compare these nuclei with these of a cell
close to the average size as found in glioblastomas. The next ob-

servation shows a giant cell with two groups of nuclei at opposite poles and around each group of nuclei there are a few short expansions like spikes. In this one we see a very wide expanse of cytoplasm with numerous short processes attached to this blood vessel (Fig. 5). In the next slide, there is another giant cell with very short and numerous processes. In this we can see this enormous nucleus connected with the other nuclei by what appears to be a thread of chromatin, so that the cell seems to be producing nuclei by budding. It is not amitosis, but resembles what happens in some protozoa or other lower animals which increase the number of nuclei by budding resulting in a plasmodium. The next slide shows a few capillaries in a glioblastoma and this giant cell with a few short processes attached to the wall of a blood vessel. The attachment of these cells to the blood vessels and the absence of reticulin surrounding the cells are the main characteristics helping us to distinguish these tumours with giant cells from tumours of mesodermal origin which never have this vascular attachment and produce an enormous amount of reticulin.

In summary, the metallic impregnations can be considered as an important tool for the characterization of the cell type in a neoplasm of the nervous tissue.

The methods that in our experience give best results are the following:

a) Silver oxide of *Cajal* in frozen sections of formalin-bromide fixed tissue, for the demonstration of astroglia and connective fibers.

b) *Wilder's* method for the demonstration of reticulin in tissues fixed in formalin and embedded in paraffin or celloidin.

c) Sublimate gold chloride of *Cajal,* or *Hortega's* modification for demonstration of the astroglia, in frozen sections, after fixation in formalin-bromide.

d) *Hortega's* silver carbonate in frozen sections — formalin-bromide fixed tissue — or *Penfield's* modification in formalin fixed material for the demonstration of oligodendrocytes with the method of *Grino* or *Meller* for paraffin sections.

e) The *Schultze-Gross* method for demonstration of neurofibrils in paraffin or celloidin sections and the *Bielschowsky, Gross* or the double impregnation of *Hortega* in frozen sections after fixation in formalin.

For reference see also: *Calvo, W.,* Tumores encephalomedulares, Valencia 1954.

Discussion

Dr. Zülch: Thank you very much for your interesting and impressive demonstration of the value of the metallic methods. I think we are particularly glad that you came as a representative of the Hortega school because you know both sides of the problem. As you know, some representatives of that school deny the value of any other stain but silver or metallic methods. However we are quite convinced that we need metallic impregnations just to give one more facet and it may be indeed a decisive facet of the whole picture. The paper is open to discussion. Dr. Rubinstein?

Dr. Rubinstein: I think Dr. Calvo's demonstration is a magnificent defence of the metallic stains and these are most striking pictures. I would like to make one practical suggestion here because it is true as Dr. Zülch says that these metallic stains meet with a great deal of opposition from some pathologists. The fact is that most pathologists may only have paraffin embedded tissue available. I think with your great experience, Dr. Calvo, it would be useful to us if we could have a summary of the best methods which you use for the specific impregnations of astrocytes, oligodendrogliocytes, microglia, both in frozen and also paraffin tissue, because one of the difficulties that you have to meet is the fact that many people not experienced in this method are offered a variety of techniques and have not the necessary experience to know which to apply. It would be one of the most valuable achievements of this Symposium if you could establish which are the best methods available. There are two further points I would like to raise on your paper which are germane, I think, to our discussion. I am not sure that I understood you correctly, but you showed in your very beautiful pictures, images of glioblastomas which we never see in normal preparations and the processes are seen much better in your silver preparations than in ordinary methods. I wonder therefore whether this does not show that some of the monstrocellular tumours are in fact gliomas. The other point which puzzles me is that you have shown us an ependymoma with suckerfeet on the blood vessel wall. As far as I remember this was the original criterion of distinction of Bailey's original paper on astroblastomas. He said that both astroblastoma and ependymoma are very similar in appearance and one of the major distinctions was that whereas the ependymoma ends up with a single process — but not suckerfeet — directed to a single point on the blood vessel, the astroblastoma has in fact this expansion. Are we entitled to call a tumour which shows suckerfeet attached to the vessels an ependymoma?

Dr. Zülch: Well, I think, as far as I remember, Bailey's description of the ependymoblastoma actually had suckerfeet because these were epithelial processes which ended with their footplate on the vessel. You remember that we originally made this distinction between ependymoma and ependymoblastoma. The ependymoma where you could show vascular processes only with phosphor-tungstic or some other methods as aniline blue-orange G, and the ependymoblastoma where you could see them already in H-E stains. Later on Bailey dropped this distinction because from the biological standpoint there was no significant difference between those groups and I don't know if Bailey has so much stressed the end-plates.

Dr. Rubinstein: I think he did.

Dr. Zülch: Yes, in the very beginning, but later on I am not quite sure about this. But we can look it up in his original book.

Dr. Rubinstein: This is important for our understanding of differences in classification. I believe this may be the reason why you would interpret some of Bailey's astroblastomas as ependymomas.

Dr. Zülch: Of his not. I think, Bailey's astroblastomas are partly astrocytomas with a particular astroblastic architecture, — these are true astroblastomas in the strict sense of the word — and some of them are definite glioblastomas with astroblastic formations, and formerly we have shown how they can arise subpially or anywhere else, i. e. near the ventricles. So I think by the end he cannot have stressed this question so much, because he dropped the astroblastoma almost entirely, but perhaps you can comment on this, Dr. Calvo.

Dr. Calvo: With respect to the first question I think that the main problem of interpretation of our cases is that we apply different techniques to the tumours. Hortega himself was against using many techniques for the same tumour or the same collection of tumours. He said that even the worst technique applied consistently to a series of tumours gave you more information than many techniques.

Dr. Zülch: May I make the suggestion that you perhaps give us a little paper telling us about the best standard methods for frozen tissue for the majority of tumours and this will be typewritten and given to the participants at the end.

Dr. Calvo: I would like to mention one thing here already because I consider this very important for the future investigations. The metallic impregnations are important for the characterisation of the cell type in a neoplasm. The methods that in our experience give best results are 1. the silver oxide of Cajal in frozen sections of formalin bromide fixed tissue for demonstration of cells and fibres, 2. the method of Wilder for reticulin in tissue fixed in formalin and in paraffin or celloidin, 3. the use of gold sublimate-chloride of Cajal or the modification of Hortega for the characterisation of astrocytes, 4. the use of silver carbonate of Hortega in frozen sections or the modification of Penfield in paraffin sections as well as the method of Grino for paraffin sections for the characterisation of oligodendrocytes, 5. the use of Schultze-Gross method for paraffin or celloidin sections or the Bielschowsky-Gross impregnation in frozen sections or formalin fixed material for demonstration of neurofibrils. If we have to choose only two I suggest the silver oxide of Cajal in frozen section and the phosphotungstic acid-haematoxylin of Mallory for paraffin sections and for any special case, as I have already mentioned, the sublimate gold chloride in order to know which are real astrocytes and also in order to know if the astrocytes are reactive or neoplastic because the reactive astrocyte is much more strongly stained.

Dr. Zülch: And for the oligodendrocyte.

Dr. Calvo: This is a special problem in paraffin sections.

Dr. Zülch: Yes, we have seen that, when your former co-worker, Dr. Meller, has prepared in our Institute some beautiful preparations of oligodendroglia in paraffin sections and I have stressed this particularly in the last 2 months because those of you who get material from outside usually get either now old formalin fixed material which is more than 2 weeks old or you get a paraffin block or a few slides and then you have to make a diagnosis.

Dr. Calvo: All the cells of the ependymoma of the glial type have these ex- of ependymomas and astroblastomas. I think that here we are dealing with a tumour that initially originated in the ependymal layer. These cells are real neuroepithelial cells with two poles, one is the epithelial and the other the glial ending. The exaggeration of either of these two poles can give us the characteristics of the neuroepithelial or the glial type of tumour. The exaggerations of the glial type loosing contact with the surface could be a parallel to what we can see in carcinoma or in an epithelioma with the cells grown far from the surface and penetrating in the connective tissue. Now, there are tumours growing deep in the brain tissue which are either the cellular type of ependymomas or the true isomorphous glioblastoma of Hortega. If these tumours grow slowly they may have time enough to develop a thicker expansion directed to the blood vessel which we always see as a glial space in haematoxylin preparations but is demonstrated by phophotungstic acid-haematoxylin or by silver impregnations. If these cells have grown there a longer time before reproducing themselves they may develop not only thicker suckerfeet but also a few short expansions at the opposite pole so they look like astroblasts and this is the normal way in which we may see the developing of the glial cells in the embryo.

Dr. Zülch: Thank you. Any other comments? Dr. Ringertz, I am sorry, I forgot you.

Dr. Ringertz: I would like to say a word about these occasional cells with suckerfeet in the ependymoma. In my opinion they can rather often be demonstrated in the cellular type of ependymoma, but I have looked upon them as astrocytes, because in my opinion there is no ependymoma which is purely monomorphic from the cellular point of view.

Dr. Calvo: All the cells of the ependymoma of the glial type have these expansions to the blood vessel. The fact that we cannot stain them with silver or phosphotungstic acid-haematoxylin or haematoxylin and eosin depends only on the size and age of these expansions, but all of them have very delicate expansions and these produce the space around the blood vessel.

Dr. Zülch: Thank you. Dr. Müller?

Dr. Müller: I ask Dr. Calvo to comment on the specificity of the metallic impregnations methods.

Dr. Calvo: This problem bears on the connection of metallic impregnation with histochemistry. It mainly depends on the presence of some substance in the cell that is argentophilic.

Dr. Sayre: I would like to ask a question for my own information. Are we sure that the metabolism of tumour cells is the same as the mature cell, because a malignant cell has a modified type of metabolism. Are we sure that because the adult cell stains with a particular silver method or gold method that the malignant cell is going always to maintain that type of staining with that particular silver or gold method as well, or could a particular cell that started with one type of staining reaction, because of its abnormal metabolism in becoming a tumour cell, pick up another type of staining with one of the metals.

Dr. Calvo: The more mature cells that are more dense, may have more protein. So it would be easier to stain those cells with any method, even the hyalin expansions of the gemistocytic astrocytes can be easily shown with eosin. The cells of the more malignant tumours which are less dense in substances may be richer in water or they may have a smaller concentration of protein, so it is more difficult to stain them. I think this is a very interesting field to study the correlation of their argentophilia, aureophilia with some histochemical methods.

Dr. Sayre: Is it not true that in photography the problem of granular participation in film depends not only on the chemical stucture but also apparently on the physical structure and that in the process of a new growth of cells there may be a change in the granular structure such that it picks up a different material.

Dr. Calvo: But what we really do with the silver impregnation is to apply silver to a preexisting structure and wash the silver from the surrounding tissue. And then we develop, we reduce this silver into granules and then develop like any film and any picture.

Dr. Zülch: Thank you, Dr. Sayre and Dr. Calvo. Would you like to ask a question, Dr. Liss?

Dr. Liss: If I may add something to Dr. Calvo's answer. We have used in our institute quite extensively silver methods and as far as specificity is concerned the oligodendroglia-technique is excellent for normal and pathological changes in the oligodendroglia. But it is not good for oligodendrogliomas. Also the astroglia-technique. It was excellent for all forms of reactive or normal astrocytes, but it will not stain astrocytomas properly but for this as a rule we used the triple technique of Hortega. And this gave us much better results. So the specificy for normal cells is not the same as for the neoplastic elements. These were at least our experiences.

Dr. Zülch: Would you like to comment, Dr. Calvo, on this?

Dr. Calvo: To force the staining procedure has an advantage and a disadvantage. You see more things but then you are not sure on the specificity. Then you have to go to the morphology. If these cells look like the normal cells we may call them oligodendrocytes or astrocytes. I think that if you force the distinction then you have to rely on something else, and one of the main features will be the relation of the cells to blood vessels. An oligodendrocyte should never show vascular feet and an astrocyte, astroblast or glioblast will show a clear relation to the blood vessels if there is a blood vessel around.

Dr. Zülch: I think, Dr. Calvo has raised a very important point, I mean, it is not only the positive or negative reaction to any specific method but it is the form as well which we have to consider. Both have to be considered because the technique depends to some extent on the skill of your technician and the material. There has been a lot of arguing about the specificity of methods. I mentioned a few remarks in my paper with Milhaud *.

Dr. Müller: May I point to the experience recently obtained with metallic impregnation in comparison with interference microscopy. By this method we can determine the density of mass in a cell and you can see that normal astrocytes have a different density from tumour astrocytes.

Dr. Calvo: I think that it would be very profitable to work at the borderland between the different methods and correlate them and see how they correspond. Electronmicroscopy, histochemistry, silver techniques. One of the most interesting sequelae of this Symposium could be such a team.

Dr. Zülch: For the night session on the microscope I suggest demonstrating all cases mentioned in the day's papers and in particular

1. Dr. Schiefer's neuroblastoma of the subfrontal olfactory region and the experimental tumour with the mesodermal component of giant perivascular cells.

2. Dr. Luginbühl's case of possible ependymoma with rosettes.

3. Dr. Calvo's case of giant cell glioma which aroused the interest of Dr. Netsky. Also his cases of spongioblastoma in comparison.

---

* *Zülch, K. J.,* and *M. Milhaud,* Etude de la fibre du neurinome, son origine schwannienne et sa nature neurectodermique. Rev. neurol. *103* (1960), 541—555.

II. The Malignancy and Grading of Tumors

The System of Grading of Gliomas

By

G. P. Sayre

In this discussion of grading of tumors of the central nervous system, I would like to confine my remarks to three phases of the problem. F i r s t, the historical background of grading of tumors; s e c o n d, the use of such a system as applied to gliomas in the central nervous system; and t h i r d, to discuss some of the criticisms that have arisen since the publication of the method of grading.

Historical Background of the Grading of Tumors

The initial idea of dividing tumors of the same type into different grades of malignancy was conceived by Dr. *A. C. Broders* [1], *a* surgical pathologist, in 1915, and his first report was published in 1920. This classification was based on an examination of 1,628 epitheliomas. This was a purely histologic classification, performed without reference to the clinical records. In reviewing this large series, it was evident that there were considerable similarities and, at the same time, differences between the tumors. On the basis of the similarities, the tumors were found to be divisible into four groups of differing degrees of cellular anaplasia. Following the suggestion of *Hansemann* that tumors were derived by dedifferentiation or anaplasia of mature cells, the degree of dedifferentiation was used as the criterion for the different categories.

The choice of dividing the groups into four grades has an interesting background. Although it is possible to group them into the usual comparative of three, as is present in all languages, such as slightly malignant, malignant and very malignant, *Broders* chose to group them into *four* grades or categories. In this he was perhaps influenced by a contemporary of his, Dr. *Henry Plummer,* whose search for an objective system of analyzing clinical symptoms and signs of thyroid disease, introduced a method of mathematical recording by grades. *Plummer* chose a basis of four grades since it was mathematically simpler to transpose a series of figures from four grades into 25 percentile groups and vice versa. In this he was a forerunner of the current specialty of biometrics. *Plummer's* influence has spread to many areas of clinical medicine and pathology at the Mayo Clinic

In *Broder's* original report he stated that if about three-fourths of the structure of the tumor was differentiated and one-fourth undifferentiated, it was graded I; if equally differentiated and undifferentiated, grade II; if three-fourths undifferentiated, grade III; and if there was no tendency for the cells to differentiate, it was grade IV. The criteria for grading was based on the character of the cells and the frequency of mitosis.

Only after having analyzed the tumors on the purely *histologic* basis did *Broders* review the clinical records of the patients. He found that of 880 cases who were operated upon and survived the immediate postoperative period, good results were obtained in 90 per cent of patients with grade I tumors, in 62 per cent of patients with grade II tumors, while only 24 per cent of patients with grade III tumors had good results; and with grade IV tumors good results occurred in only 10 per cent. Thus the histologic grading was borne out by the biological results.

Unfortunately, certain word usages have led to some confusion in these studies and *Broders* clarified his statements in an article written in 1926 [2], in this paper he placed the emphasis on degrees of undifferentiation or anaplasia or self control of *all* of the cells. rather than on the percentage of undifferentiated tumor cells, for the basis of grading. Thus he defined grade I tumors as those containing cells in which differentiation or self-control ranges from almost 100 per cent to 75 per cent and undifferentiation from 0 to 25 per cent; grade II should represent a carcinoma in which differentiation or self-control ranges from 75 to 50 per cent, grade III represents carcinoma in which differentiation ranges from 50 to 25 per cent, grade IV represents carcinoma in which differentiation or self-control ranges from 25 per cent to practically 0, and undifferentiation from 75 to about 100 per cent. In other words, the tumors were classified according to the degree of dedifferentiation or anaplasia *of all the cells* rather than on a percentage of dedifferentiated cells, since in many cases the cells were uniformly dedifferentiated while the *degree* of dedifferentiation varied between the different tumors.

This method has been the basis for the extensive use of a system of grading of tumors of all types, as used by pathologists at the Mayo Clinic, and it is applied to all tumors of the body. Modifications and refinements of the criteria of dedifferentiation have occurred over the years, based on reviews of histopathologic material as sufficient numbers of cases have been obtained, but the same essential *histologic* criteria have been used and with the same general relationship of histologic grading to prognosis. It should be *emphasized* that by no manner of means does the total number of tumors of any organ fall into four equal-sized compartments. Thus most carcinomas of the stomach fall into grades III and IV, while most cancers of the colon fall into grades I and II; it is the *appearance* of the cells which determines the grade.

The Use of Grading as Applied to Tumors of the Central Nervous System

The development of a system of grading of tumors of the central nervous system was delayed long after the usefulness of this system had been demonstrated in tumors elswhere in the body for two main reasons. First, was the requirement of accumulating a significant number of gliomas of the different types which could be graded, and the grading correlated with the clinical course. Second, was the natural reluctance to substitute a new classification for the well accepted system of *Bailey* and *Cushing* [3]. The first requirement was not fully met until 1949, although a tentative grading system was instituted in 1938. In 1949 there were available for study biopsies of tumors of the astrocytoma group from 161 patients who survived at least one month after operation, and 57 biopsies of similar patients with ependymomas. For the practical details of the system of grading of these tumors and the oligodendrogliomas, I must refer you to the original articles of *Svien, Mabon, Kernohan* [4], and to the fascicle of "Tumors of the Central Nervous System" [5] and the chapter on "Pathology of Malignant Tumors, Central and Peripheral Nervous System" [6] published by Butterworth and Company of London. Suffice it to say that because of the rather complex nature of the tumors, the term dedifferentiation refers to the character of the cell, the nuclei, the cytoplasm, the cytoplasmic processes, the number of bizarre and multinucleated cells, the frequency of mitoses, the vascular changes and the degree of degeneration.

The theoretical problem of introducing a new classification to supplant that introduced by *Bailey* and *Cushing* was naturally a formidable one, since the classification has been so widely accepted. But this classification was admittedly tentative. Essentially this classification was an attempt to designate a tumor according to its resemblance to a cell in the embryological development of the brain, as this was then understood. The hypotheses of *Cohnheim* [7] and *Ribbert* [8] that tumors arose from cell rests, did in fact lead to this method of classification and this was satisfactory for the more malignant tumors with a fancied resemblance to embryonic cells. But *Bailey* and *Cushing* found it necessary to use the theory of *Samuel:* that the least differentiated cells were more easily capable of forming tumors, to account for the development of some of the more mature tumors. The authors were admittedly dismayed to note that the indifferent cells of Schaper, which they had originally planned to use as the source of many mature tumors, were, in reality, adult cells, as discovered by *Del Rio Hortega* and classified by him as mature oligodendroglia and mature microglia. The great stumbling block was, and still is, in the Bailey-Cushing classification, how to account for the tumors originally called spongioblastoma multiforme. Here it is instructive to note that in their monograph *Bailey* and *Cushing* suggested the possibility that these tumors could be derived from protoplasmic astrocytes, since in several cases of multiple operations there was a change from the histologic appearance of protoplasmic astrocytes to typical spongioblastoma multiforme with numerous mitoses. In each case a dedifferentiation seems to have occurred with a corresponding increase in the rapidity of growth. So convinced were they of the correctness of the theories of *Cohnheim* and *Ribbert,* however, that, although no such cell had been described by the embryologist, they manufactured one, the glioblast, to account for the common highly malignant tumor of the brain where this transformation could not be identified.

Although the *Bailey* and *Cushing* classification was originally described as tentative, its obvious advantages of bringing some order out of the chaos of previous descriptions was of immediate value, intensified by the apparent clinical correlation that the more *embryonic appearing* the tumor the more rapid its growth.

Meanwhile there had been a considerably different approach to tumor histogenesis in the fields of general pathology, which had been ignored by most neuropathologists. The common theory of cell rests as the etiology of tumors had never been taken too seriously by the pathologists. Rather it was early recognized that the tumors develop, for the most part, from some disturbance in adult cells. The exceptions were mainly those tumors found in infancy and childhood, many being found at or shortly after birth, or those of a teratomatous nature. This concept of the development of tumors from disturbed *adult tissue growth* and a realization that new growth or tissue arose de novo, not by reversal of cells to embryologic forms, was manifest in the many examples of tumors produced by external means, beginning with the chimney sweep's cancer of the scrotum. This stand was progressively supported by first, the production, both undesired and desired, of tumors by radiation; and later by the investigations of the hydrocarbon carcinogens, notably by *Kennaway* [9] and associates.

That not all of the neuropathologists in the twenties were subservient to the ideas of *Cohnheim* is indicated by the classifications of *Roussy, Cornil* and *Lhermitte* and of *Cox. Bailey,* with the availability of new cases, modified his own classification in 1933, as did *Cushing* and *Penfield.* Only *Globus,* who with *Strauss,* had been one of the earliest exponents of the *Cohnheim* and *Ribbert* theories, maintained to the end the embryologic classification; in his last article in 1953 with *Carres, Globus* stoutly maintained his original position of 1925. Probably the greatest inconoclast of all was *Scherer,* who castigated *Ribbert* and his fellow neuropathologists in language hardly seen before or since. Unfortunately his own method of classification is also extremely complex and requires study of the whole intact tumor, particularly the growing edges.

In the years following the initial publication of the original classification of *Kernohan* in 1949, less and less emphasis has been placed on the ideas of *Cohnheim* and *Ribbert,* with the exception of *Globus* mentioned above, and more and more acceptance, in greater or lesser degrees, of the ideas of dedifferentiation has occurred. (Amongst the distinguished authors are Drs. *Calvo, Ringertz* and our chairman, Dr. *Zülch.*) The classifications more recently proposed, however, still usually include the glioblastoma multiforme, but usually out of inertia or sentimental reasons. The term does not designate a very well-understood tumor histologically, and as I will mention later, there is really no need to separate this tumor into an independent group.

The areas of criticism of the system of grading have fallen into several categories. I will try to group them and attempt to answer the criticisms where possible, and at the same time point out the well-defined limitations of the method.

The common complaint has been that the system of grading is artificial; that is, that to attempt to count the number of differentiated cells and then to find the percentage of undifferentiated cells so as to place the tumor in a certain grade is inexact because of the variability of the tumor cells. I believe those who have taken this stand have misread the criteria listed for grading. As pointed out previously, the system of grading takes into consideration the *overall* picture of the tumor in *all* its manifestations. The grading is determined on the basis of the deviation of the cells from the normal, the degree of dedifferentiation present. Naturally, if one part of the tumor is well differentiated and another less differentiated, the tumor is graded on the basis of the least differentiated part.

Because some tumors have different appearances in different areas the question has been asked "How is it possible to grade the tumor — how can one know that the tumor is homogenous?" This question was asked particularly by *Scherer* concerning every proposed method of classification. I can only answer the question by stating that any pathologist is faced with the same problem no matter what method of classification is used. No histopathologic examination is better than the method of sampling. That the hazards of such misclassification due to sampling may be disastrous as far as the care of the individual patient is concerned is certainly *not* borne out, since, in repeated cases classified under any system, the actual designation of the tumor type has been followed by fairly consistent results as far as the growth of the tumor is concerned.

At this point, it is pertinent to state that the theory of grading by the degree of dedifferentiation does not assume that in the development of a tumor, the cells gradually change from a normal cell to a slightly malignant cell then a more malignant and finally a very malignant cell. Whatever it is that produces the malignant change may affect the cells at the very beginning, so that the alteration is complete in the first series of cell divisions, and the manner of growth is determined by the altered metabolism at that time. In examining highly malignant tumors of epithelial or glandular structures which are small in size, it is the usual experience to see a sudden alteration of the cells without any transitional zone, or the zone may be limited to a few cells only. This is easily recognized in highly malignant, grade IV carcinomas of the stomach, where highly malignant cells may be present within the areas of the normal epithelial lining, and without evidence of gradual transformation. Even when there is evidence of mixed growth of cells in a tumor, such as in so-called mixed astrocytoma and secondary glioblastoma, are we really justified in saying the glioblastoma originated from the astrocytoma? Certainly the reverse is well documented in the field of general pathology. For example, highly malignant squamous cell carcinomas may have multiple foci of cell keratinization in the center of nodules, while the peripheral areas consist of extremely anaplastic cells. The course of the tumor is determined and the prognosis correlates with the areas of least differentiation. To account for this histologic picture, it has been suggested that the highly dedifferentiated cells that make up the most malignant portion of the tumor tend to differentiate to the more normal structure. In the process of the metabolism of the individual tumor cell attempts are made to progress to the differentiated stage, forming the central area of cell keratinization, the so-called pearly bodies of malignant epitheliomas.

A further criticism is based on the assumption that the grading of a tumor leads to a false sense of security by the surgeon. The system of grading, however, refers only to the histologic appearance of the tumor; it does *not* refer to the size or location of the tumor. In this, however, the classification by grading does not differ from the classifications of *Bailey* and *Cushing,* or of *Roussy* and *Oberling,* or of most others. A grade I subependymal astrocytoma of the aqueduct may be more immediately lethal when it reaches a certain size than a grade IV astrocytoma of the temporal lobe which can be removed en bloc. In a similar vein, the system of grading of cancer of the stomach has been challenged by others because it does not take into consideration the spread of the tumor. Thus *Dukes* has proposed the classification of such tumors into types A, B, C, wherein type A refers to tumors limited to the mucosa, type B, tumors extending to involve the serosa and type C when lymph node metastases are found. *Dukes* found the prognosis to be consistently worse as the type changed from A to C, and with a large series, this method appeared almost as valuable as the method of grading. But obviously, these criteria cannot be compared — one refers to cell metabolism, the other to cell localization. Cell localization is, of course, extremely important. *Dochat* reviewed a series of tumors of the stomach in which he both graded the tumors on the basis of cell metabolism and typed them on the basis of location according to *Duke*'s method. The combined information was more accurate than either method alone as far as prognosis was concerned, as might logically be expected. The similar use of *both* a method of histologic grading and tumor localization in the central nervous system would certainly be of great value to the neurosurgeon.

In the classification of gliomas, not all tumors are classifiable. Most noticeable in this group are the medulloblastomas, which in this classification are placed in a single separate category. However, in any review of a large series of these tumors, there are different cell types and manners of growth. As yet, no successful method has been determined, to my knowledge, to differentiate these tumors and subdivide them. As to the more bizarre tumors, one can gain some insight into their biological behavior even if one has no assurance of the cell types, by using the same method for grading the unknown cells. As more work is done on these tumors, some will be classified as members of the glioma group, others, as for example the so-called giant cell glioblastomas will be recognized as giant cell sarcomas. The essential course of the tumors depends on the cell metabolism, not the site of origin, but the course of the patient depends in part on the location of the tumor.

Finally, as far as the question as to whether tumors are ever derived from embryonic cells, I believe that there is good evidence to the effect that certain types of tumors may well be derived from the cells before full adult development of the cells of the brain have occurred. This is most probable in the cases of the medulloblastomas, or at least in some of them, which seem definitely to have originated from the external granular layer of the cerebellum. But in addition to this, there are certainly other tumors found in the neonatal period which have probably originated before full adult differentiation has occurred within the cells of the brain. Similar tumors of peculiar type are found in other areas of the body, particularly the Wilm's [9] tumor of the kidney and the peculiar retroperitoneal tumors of infants, and thus there is precedence for such tumor derivation.

In conclusion, let me reiterate certain points.

1. The method of grading of tumors is based on the histologic appearance of the tumor, not on its position.

2. The features upon which the grading depends include the whole histologic appearance of the tumor; that is, the tumor cell including its nucleus, nucleolus, and cytoplasm, and the reaction of the blood vessels and surrounding tissues to the tumor, and their interrelationships. The emphasis is placed on the degree of deviation from the normal.

3. With few exceptions, notably the medulloblastomas, tumors are derived by anaplasia or dedifferentiation from adult cells, brought about by an unknown cause or, more probably, multiple causes. With this understanding, it brings the tumors of the glial group within the same biological disturbance as tumors in other parts of the body.

References

1. *Broders, A. C.*, Sqamous Cell Epithelioma of the Lip: A Study of Five Hundred and thirty-seven Cases. J. A. M. A. 74 (1920), 656—664. — 2. *Broders, A. C.*, The Grading of Carcinoma. Minnesota Med. 8 (1925), 76—730. — 3. *Bailey, P.*, and *H. Cushing*, A Classification of the Tumors of the Glioma Group on a Histogenetic Basis with a Correlated Study of Prognosis. Philadelphia: The J. B. Lippincott Company. 1926. — 4. *Kernohan, J. W., R. F. Mabon, H. J. Svien*, and *A. W. Adson*, A Simplified Classification of Gliomas. Proc. Staff Meet. Mayo Clin. 24 (1949), 71—75. — 5. *Kernohan, J. W.*, and *G. P. Sayre*, Tumors of the Central Nervous System. Atlas of Tumors Pathology Section X, Fascicles 35

and 37. Washington, D. C., Armed Forces Institute of Pathology. 1952. — 6. *Kerno-han, J. W.*, and *G. P. Sayre*, In: Cancer, Raven, R. W., Editor, pp. 525—551. London, Butterworth & Co. 1958. — 7. *Cohnheim, J.*, Lectures on General Pathology: A Handbook for Practitioners and Students. (Translated from the Second German Edition by A. B. McKee.) London: The New Sydenham Society. *2* (1889), 746—821. — 8. *Ribbert, H.*, Quoted by Scherer. — 9. *Kennaway, E. L.*, Experiments on Cancer Producing Substances. Brit. Med. J. *2* (1925), 1—4. — 10. *Roussy, G.*, and *C. Oberling*, Les Tumeurs des Centres Nerveux et des Nerfs Peripheriques Paris: Atlas du Cancer, Fascicles 9 et 10. Alcon. 1931. — 11. *Cox, L. B.*, Observations Upon the Nature of Rate of Growth and Operability of the Intracranial Tumors Derived from 135 Patients. Med. J. Australia *1* (1934), 182—196. — 12. *Bailey, P.*, Histologic Diagnosis of Tumors of the Brain. Arch. Neurol. Psychiatr., London, *27* (1932), 1290—1297. — 13. *Cushing, H.*, Intracranial Tumors. Springfield and Baltimore: C. C. Thomas & Co. 1932. — 14. *Penfield, W.*, The Classification of Gliomas. Arch. Neurol. Psychiatr., London, *26* (1931), 745—753. — 15. *Globus, J. H.*, and *I. Strauss*, Spongioblastoma Multiforme. Arch. Neurol. Psychiatr. *14* (1925), 139—191. — 16. *Globus, J. H.*, and *R. M. Cares*, Neuroepithelioma. Its Place in Histogenetic Classification of Primary Neuroectodermal Brain Tumors. J. Neuropath., Baltimore, *12* (1953), 311—348. — 17. *Scherer, H. J.*, Critical Review of Pathology of Cerebral Gliomas. J. Neurol., London, *3* (1940), 147—177. — 18. *Calvo, W.*, Tumores Encefalomedulares. V Supplement, Archivo españ. morf. 1954. — 19. *Ringertz, N.*, "Grading" of Gliomas. Acta path. microbiol., Scand. *27* (1950), 51—64. — 20. *Zülch, K. J.*, The Present State of the Classification of Intracranial Tumour and Its Value for the Neurosurgeon. Rev. brasil. cir. *40* (1960), 247—264. In: *Fields* and *Sharkey* and coll., The Biology and Treatment of Intracranial Tumors. Chapter VII, p. 157—177. Ch. C. Thomas Publ., Springfield, Ill., 1962. — 21. *Dukes, C. E.*, The Classification of Cancer of the Rectum. J. Path. Bact. *3* (1932), 323—332. — 22. *Dochat, G. R.*, A Prognostic Comparison of Serosal and Nodal Spread in Carcinoma of the Stomach with Classification into Duke's Types. Thesis Univ. of Minn. 1941.

Discussion

Dr. Zülch: Thank you Dr. Sayre. Your contribution gave us very remarkable correlations with general pathologic problems, which I think will be particularly valuable for the discussion. Since the only of our group who has particularly discussed grading has been Dr. Ringertz I beg you to tell us your concept of grading.

Dr. Ringertz: I will give a little historical data. It was during the time that I was neuropathologist to Dr. Olivecrona late in the fourties, that the surgeons often asked me, whether I could not say something more prognostically. "You say this is an astrocytoma and in several cases you are doubtful, the tumour could be malignant, could you be a little more definite." Then I decided to create criteria, for what I though should be an "intermediate" group, tumours which seemed not quite benign astrocytomas but on the other hand which I would not frankly diagnose as malignant gliomas. And thus I happened to work out a grading system for the astrocytomas quite on my own without influence by any other pathologist's conception and I gave a little paper on that in 1946 at a Norwegian Neurosurgical Meeting. And then when I saw the report of a Symposium at the Mayo Clinic in February 1949 I thought it was desirable

to put my system forward and to compare my results with those of the Mayo
Clinic just to find out if their system was more satisfactory than my own based
on the biological features of those tumours which I had graded histologically *.
Now when you make a comparison on biological properties using such criteria
as postoperative survival it is naturally of the utmost importance that you only
compare groups of brain tumours that could be compared that is to say for
these tumours it is the hemisphere gliomas, You can't put in the central gliomas
in this comparison because there are certain factors operating which may result
in a poor survival time. It was rather simple with the astrocytomas which I felt
could be quite easily divided into three groups, benign, an intermediate group
and a malignant group for which I used the name glioblastoma. But when we
then came to the other kinds of gliomas according to Bailey/Cushing's scheme,
the ependymomas and the oligodendrogliomas the matter was more complicated
because it was quite possible to discern some tumours which were structurally
easy to recognize as ependymomas or oligodendrogliomas but where the cellular
make up made you as a general pathologist say that this tumour was moderately
anaplastic and where there were mitoses and where you could suspect that it
would be a more rapidly growing tumour than the bulk of those tumours with
their benign appearance. But then, if you looked up the biological course of these
cases you found that they did have a characteristic survival time, and preoperative periods, a little higher age incidence etc. But the difference was not
very marked; for instance not at all so marked as between astrocytoma and
frank glioblastoma. I should say that among these oligos and ependymomas
several could be histologically recognized because of their malignant appearance,
these compared biologically very well with my intermediate group of astrocytomas in the series astrocytoma — glioblastoma. Then when you are looking
upon the great mass of glioblastomas you find specimens in which you can
discern here and there a small area with traces of an ependymomalike structure,
but anaplastic and distorted, but you can still recognize it with classical stains
and you may feel more convinced if you have made any silver impregnations
and so on. And as to the oligodendrogliomas it is much more difficult. These
glioblastomas with traces of ependymal structure have been described before.
Among the oligos I have not seen any author who has said these isomorphic
glioblastomas should be malignant oligodendrogliomas. But after all that is
theoretically possible. So when I thought it would be possible to go on with
a three step grading in the case of ependymomas and oligodendrogliomas I found
that it would be possible to identify the benign and intermediate group but no
further, because although you could in some cases suspect that a glioblastoma
was a malignant ependymoma or oligodendroglioma, I did not find it satisfactory to use the grading in these further steps. Thus the term glioblastoma
implied this malignant glial tumour upon which theoretically at least the three
big families of benign tumours converge when they go anaplastic. Therefore my
schema was to have the astrocytoma, — benign astrocytoma-intermediate group,
oligodendroglioma — malignant oligodendroglioma, if you want to call it that
way, but better "intermediate group" and ependymoma, intermediate group etc.
Then we have as a common group glioblastoma this being the frankly malignant
counterpart of all these three varieties of benign glioma. It was possible to compare my figures and those given by the Mayo Clinic pathologists. This is of value
because it seems that my group glioblastoma with a percentage of 56% is very

---

* *Ringertz, N.*, "Grading" of gliomas. Acta path. microbiol. Scand. 27 (1950),
51—64.

comparable. In the age of the patients there is a gradual rising when you
come to the more malignant stages in both material. The preoperative duration
is naturally something very unreliable. Postoperative survival is more reliable
because both the Mayo and my material were made up of hemisphere gliomas,
but may I ask Dr. Sayre if there cerebellar astrocytomas were included in his
material?

Dr. Sayre: Some of them were, yes.

Dr. Ringertz: Then my material is not very comparable because mine contained only cerebral not the cerebellar forms. Apart from astrocytomas, I tried to
apply my grading system to our ependymoma material and compare it with
that of the Mayo Clinic. When I looked through my material classed as glioblastoma I found about 9 or 10 cases, which I thought had traces of ependymal
structure and I put them in the same intermediate group because I wanted
to compare my figures with those of the Mayo Clinic. Now it seems to me that
my intermediate group here certainly includes 7 ependymomas but with that
malignant rather anaplastic cell picture it is not quite as large as the same
group in the Mayo grading, so perhaps I have been rather restrictive in finding
the signs of anaplasia. When we come to the average of postoperative survival,
it compares very well at least with the first three groups of the Mayo Clinic.
So I am convinced that when I grade ependymomas into the benign and well
recognized and the rather anaplastic and finally glioblastomas with traces of
ependymal structure that it compares very well at least with the first three
grades of the Mayo Clinic grading. I was also able to give some figures on oligodendrogliomas but I did not dare to include probable oligodendrogliomas
among the glioblastomas because it was very difficult to find out which you
admit in that group. But there is no similar grading of oligodendrogliomas in
the Mayo Clinic Proceedings of that time or later. But I want to make clear
here that if a well recognized tumour is an oligodendroglioma with a rather malignant anaplastic cellular pattern, it still has a prognosis of 64 for the benign and
47 postoperative months for the malignant types. Therefore we can recognize
a tumour as oligodendroglioma but if we find it malignant it should be included
in an intermediate group. Now I have found that grading of tumours is something which is regarded as a service which the pathologist gives the clinician.
It is of practical value. But it has not very much to do with the real scientific
classification of tumours. So a grading system could be grafted on the diagnosis
list if it could be internationally agreed upon, but only if the grades are so very
clear that you can apply them without difficulty. It is not enough to put a case
into a list of tumours called so and so when that grade does not make sense
because the pathologist in the remotest part of the world can't follow the criteria.

Dr. Zülch: We are all glad to have this report from you because it shows
that at quite another place, far away from the Mayo Clinic the same idea has
been developed, and that by influence of your position as a general pathologist
and with the education of a general pathologist the concept has been the same
and I should say the conclusions are the same, only the technique differs somewhat. This technique of grading may be perhaps the starting point of our discussion, because we all will, I am sure, agree on the necessity of grading
malignancy somehow as pathologists have always done. It is only the concept
of technique which differs, and I may just stress this difference which seems
to me to be the starting point for the divergence of the various concepts. That
is, the principle underlying the Mayo group is that every well defined tumour
group has its four grades (apart from medulloblastomas) whereas some other
people say that these four grades are not present in every group and that

the groups have so to speak a grade of their own and we only have to fix the
various grades within these groups. Later on I may come back to this discussion;
the two papers are now open for discussion. I know that Dr. Woolf has
something to say on grading.

Dr. Woolf: I do not think I have anything very definite to say, but if one is
going to grade neoplasms I do think it would be valuable to the surgeon if when
we said a tumour had a certain grade it meant the same thing whatever series
of tumours was concerned. I think if the survival period of the grade 2 astrocytoma is only two thirds of the survival period of the grade 2 ependymoma
unless the surgeon has taken very great care to read all that has been written
about grading he is going to get a misconception and I would only say that if
it were possible to have some sort of a grading system in which the numbers
of the grades meant the same whatever the series of the tumour that might be
more valuable.

Dr. Ringertz: Not only if in the nervous system tumours but all over pathology
tumours have the same grading systems. Then I think that my 3 steps of grading
is actually remaining on the Broder's system because the trend is in various
tumours, in uterine tumours and in many kinds of tumours to devise a benign
group and a intermediate group and a frankly malignant group.

Dr. Zülch: This is the old traditional and very well based concept of general
pathology which has always included an intermediate group "semibenign" or
"semimalignant" between the benign and malignant tumours.

Dr. Sayre: I would like to say that as far as comparison is concerned a system
of 4 groups is an improvement as it comprises a relatively benign group together
with three groups of slightly malignant, more malignant and most malignant
tumours. Willis who in his books condemns grading as severely as most people
do that I have come in contact with, describes carcinoma of the breast as slightly
malignant, more malignant and very malignant. So he graded by three. He
contracted himself. This is to me a perpetual semantic difficulty. The only
purpose of grading in four is in when one deals with numbers of a large series.
It is much easier mathematically to divide by four than it is to divide by three,
$33^1/_3\%$ is very hard to work out. It is very easy to add a column of figures and
divide by four and have 25% of groups. This was the reason why Henry
Plummer divided things originally in degree 1—4 and we have followed this.
I have really no complaint against people who divide by 3, the old holy number,
just as Greek is in 3, Latin is in 3, German in 3, English in 3, good, better,
best, everything is in 3, but mathematically it is not practical. But I do feel
that in general the criteria do correspond very much throughout the body
whether we grade a tumour "one" in the stomach, one in the breast, one in
the uterus, grade one in the brain. The survival rates are fairly constant. It is
quite certain that in the two series described here there is a difference of percentage in the survival times between ependymomas and the astrocytomas. But
I think if one talks to the statistician this difference in this small series is not out
of line and certainly it does change when you deal with large numbers. It is
obvious that any system of grading is not a pure prognostic sign for the individual patient and this, at least, is accepted by all the neurosurgeons of the
Mayo Clinic. Two patients may have a grade 2 tumour, one of them is going
to die in 3 weeks and the other one perhaps in 3 years. And there are always
exceptions. I remember a case of a patient with a most malignant appearing
carcinoma of the thyroid. This patient should have died at the end of 6 months,
but she was still alive 5 years later. The pathologist would not change his grading
number, he said this is a biological exception. And I think that this is important

that biologically things are not mathematically clear with an absolute 100%. We have to understand that biological systems are variable. Grading is a method which works out in the larger series, but there are exceptions in the individual patients.

Dr. Zülch: Thank you, Dr. Sayre.

Dr. Netsky: Most of us probably employ forms of grading when we call a feature slight, moderate or severe. This equivalent of one, two or three would not be objectionable. But one concern I have for this system of grading in which numbers are used is that is does lend itself to a mathematical quality that you have already indicated does not exist, I think this, one of the major objections I have to using a numerical system rather than a descriptive system. But there is another approach that I would like to mention and that is, in your grading system there is a concept of the origin of tumours which I don't believe you or anyone at this table has, viz that you can tell the cell of origin of this particular tumour. I presented some experimental evidence about this problem and there is a good deal of evidence in man. Most of these gliomas are mixed and if they are not, their cells of origin are difficult to determine. Most gliomas we see have mixtures of different kinds of cells. Despite your classification, you can't identify the cell of origin of this particular tumour as an ependymal cell or an astrocytic cell. I don't think there is any scientific verification that you can do it nor indeed that it does exist in the origin of cancer.

Dr. Sayre: I would like to answer this and this is a problem in any system. What is the glioblastoma multiforme supposed to be? It is a term we use as a substitute.

Dr. Netsky: Well, we are always safer when we describe what we see rather than infer. If I say glioblastoma multiforme and I can give you a description of what I have seen I think we are understanding better. You give me a mathematical grade for a complex tissue, and I am not sure that I know what you are speaking of.

Dr. Sayre: I don't know what you mean when you say a glioblastoma multiforme except by long reading of the literature in which a glioblastoma multiforme has been described as such and such a lesion. But the term glioblast. What is a glioblast?

Dr. Netsky: It is a derived term. We don't have any such cell. The word was derived to have a name for a tumour.

Dr. Sayre: They had to bring the name out of the air because they had said it must be an embryological cell.

Dr. Zülch: Yes, but I think, this concept, this early concept was in order to get the chaos of classification out of this disorder and to get somewhere and I think Bailey himself would not stress the histogenetic derivation implied in his system.

·*Dr. Netsky:* I think also the point should be made clear that one of the motives Bailey and Cushing had in concocting the term glioblast was to avoid confusion with spongioblastoma multiforme and spongioblastoma polare. It is merely a question of words and I don't think it is an important issue.

Dr. Sayre: If the question of the word is not an important issue why is the question of grading them into four grades important?

Dr. Netsky: We have an accepted classification, perfectly useful, and not different from yours. Your classification adds nothing except more words for the same thing.

Dr. Sayre: Well, I must stand by this because I think that one must recognize that one can find in any large series of tumours a tumour which is made of cells which are easily recognizable as astrocytes, cells which have some astrocytic features, with those which have at the same time very bizarre cells and finally a group of cells which are extremely bizarre. And this is a series of quite sharp changes one from another. And there is no absolute differentiation between this tumour, the next tumour, the third tumour and the fourth. There are merely percentual variations and they are all members of the same family. When one introduces a new term — glioblastoma multiforme — to the uninitiated, this is regarded by them as a totally different tumour from the astrocytoma or the oligodendroglioma or the ependymoma. I do not believe that it is. And I disagree with Dr. Rubinstein and his book on this idea.

Dr. Zülch: Well, you see, there was a long discussion of H. J. Scherer's about primary and secondary glioblastomas and quite a good many of us including myself would think that the glioblastoma is an entirely different tumour from the astrocytoma. It is anaplastic in its origin; there are though also secondary glioblastomas, i. e. astrocytomas, where you can follow the course from a benign fibrillary hard astrocytoma grade one into a real glioblastoma with necroses and vessel proliferations and excess of stroma. But this tumour is pretty rare, it may be 5% or 10% of the astrocytomas, I don't know, but it does occur. So I would myself like Scherer always stress the point that the glioblastoma is a tumour of its own so to speak, a primary cancer of the brain, the anaplastic "cancer" of the glia, quite different from what an astrocytoma is. But let us hear Dr. Rubinstein on this topic.

Dr. Rubinstein: From this extremely interesting discussion and from the papers of Dr. Sayre and Dr. Ringertz it seems to me there are two aspects in this question of grading which are open to discussion. There is first, and I think this is the important contribution of the Mayo Clinic, the theoretical concept behind grading. This is the emphasis on anaplasia or dedifferentiation. To me the most important contribution is the emphasis on a derivation of most of these glial tumours, particularly in adults, from adult cells in opposition to the embryonic cell theory of Cohnheim and Ribbert. We would agree with the Mayo Clinic that the large majority of glioblastomas are derived from mature adult astrocytes. Therefore there is no essential difference from the concept that many glioblastomas are in your terminology grade four astrocytomas. Now I come to the second aspect of grading, the practical one, for the neurosurgical clinic. And here the question arises does it in fact work? This is its only justification in my point of view and the Mayo Clinic has put forward in their papers, a clinico-pathological correlation which they believe works. A patient with an astrocytoma grade one has a better prognosis and those of grade three and four have a poor prognosis. And here I think we come into practical difficulties. The question of sampling is of course extremely important. You get the peripheral biopsy from a superficial tumour with a relatively benign appearance which will already show dedifferentiation in the deeper parts in the corpus callosum. In a case like this grading seems to me unreliable and even misleading. Secondly there is the important question of the localisation of tumours. In these large series that the Mayo Clinic has collected for their statistical overall assessment of their prognosis the group of astrocytomas would always include of course a large number of the cerebellar ones. In these we have a much better prognosis than in the cerebral astrocytomas in adults. If you grade one, or perhaps grade two in a slightly more pleomorphic one, you are giving a good prognosis. You may also do the same on a grade one or two cerebral astrocytoma in adults. Now in these cases our feeling is that although they may appear benign at first they have a much worse prognosis than the cerebellar ones. So the value of grading would very much depend on where the tumour lies. And this to some extent weakens this statistical approach. Thirdly I think one of our great objections is that it gives to the pathologist a false claim to prognosis. You can say that at this particular moment the tumour is grade one or two, but you cannot say whether or not tomorrow, next week or in the next two or three years the tumour may not undergo dedifferentiation and anaplasia. And this element of time is the most important. We have to study the whole evolution of the tumour. And grading into one, two, three, four neglects this aspect. Then finally, you may notice in the recent literature some difficulties in the actual grading. I have read papers where people described astrocytomas as grade 2 or 3. They were not even certain where to grade them. Are we therefore to have a grade $2^1/_2$?

Dr. Sayre: I don't want to answer all of these questions but just to start off with the last one. It is quite possible to grade according to a hundred different characteristics. At the Mayo Clinic we grade things like reflexes, increased reflexes grade 1, 2, 3 and 4 and decreased reflexes grade 1 to 4. It is a simple method of giving information in papers and if you see a patient two days later you can tell whether the reflexes were increased or decreased by comparison with the initial statement. The grading of heart murmurs is done in the same way in degrees of loudness. It is purely a form of mechanism of putting a definite term in a short space period, instead of a long description of what one is dealing with. So the problem of people as to whether to grade 2 or 3 is the problem of a type of person who does not know whether to put on a black tie or a green tie. These are problems of people who cannot make up their minds and this I don't think is a fault of the system, it is the fault of the person who is doing this. Dr. Rubinstein has modified Dr. Zülch's standpoint I believe in suggesting that there are more glioblastomas derived from astrocytomas than Dr. Zülch would accept. And as I mentioned in the discussion here, in cancer of the cervix for instance we are doing biopsies and you can have a biopsy which looks fine and perfectly normal except for a minimal area which may require 25 sections to find. You may find grade 4 tumour in that cervix without a change through grades 1, 2, 3 and 4; a direct change has occured in the original metabolism of that cell. We classify according to the most malignant types of cells which are present, so the grading does not assume the fact that the tumour has to pass through the different grades to be grade 4. I think that these are factors of misunderstanding. Finally I don't think it is the duty of the pathologist to completely shoulder the problems of the neurosurgeon who is responsible as far as the care of the patients is concerned. The pathologist will give an idea of what he sees to be the biological speed of growth of the tumour. If it is in a temporal lobe, take it all out; if it is a cancer of the breast and you take it all out, the patient can live 50 years without any evidence of recurrence. If it is a grade one and she already has a metastasis this patient is going to die. The localisation of a tumour, accessibility of a tumour, the method of removal of a tumour are problems for the surgeon himself. They are not problems of the pathologist and I don't believe that we as pathologists can look into the head of a patient and say you did actually get into the tumour. This is particularly true for needle biopsies of tumours growing through the corpus callosum and involving both frontal lobes. Pathologists should not go beyond the histological appearance of a tumour and I don't believe that most pathologists would try.

Dr. Rubinstein: What information would you convey by grading?

Dr. Sayre: The information that this particular group of cells are in this particular tumour.

Dr. Rubinstein: In this particular sample.

Dr. Sayre: Yes, this is true of all pathological examinations, it is the risk of any pathological examination.

Dr. Zülch: This has nothing to do with grading, I think, here we really have to defend Dr. Sayre. It is the risk of any pathological examination to take the wrong bit and biopsy is easier naturally in great organs such as the general surgeons take out. If you have a total breast, you can cut through the whole breast, and you can even count and figure out that the tumour is 30% undifferentiated. In brain tumours you have three little bits like a finger nail. What are you going to do then because three-fifths of the tumour have gone down the sucker.

Dr. Rubinstein: This is exactly the objection to grading.

Dr. Sayre: Yes, but not only to grading but to any form of biological prognosis.

Dr. Rubinstein: Yes, I think that is why it is so much easier and so much more valuable to grade cancer of the breast or cancer of the rectum. There grading is of value, because usually the information you have from the surgical point of view is much more complete than in the brain. I have no objection to grading as such but the reservations are very important and I agree with Dr. Netsky that in fact we all do grade by reporting malignant or relatively benign tumours, but the danger here lies in giving it some sort of pseudo-scientific accuracy. You can grade carcinomas of the lip or the alimentary tract or the breast or the rectum. The question is can you safely grade gliomas in all surgical specimens?

Dr. Zülch: Well, I think, this may be one of the real dangers. It gives a semi-accuracy or a feeling of semi-accuracy to the neurosurgeon if he gets a report "grade 2" he may think himself quite safe that this is the actual prognosis whereas our prognosis is always based on much more uncertainty than that of the general pathologist in surgical specimens. This is one of the objections I have to make.

Dr. Sayre: But I cannot see the difference between this "grade 1 or 2" or if you tell the surgeon the patient has an astrocytoma, does that not indicate that you were dealing with a benign tumour?

Dr. Rubinstein: It makes a great difference if you tell the surgeon the patient has a diffuse cerebral astrocytoma with areas of anaplasia as compared with the classical circumscribed and benign cerebellar tumour. This to me is much more important and valuable information than just saying astrocytoma grade 1, 2, 3 or 4.

Dr. Sayre: The surgeon knows where the tumour came from and if he has an astrocytoma of the cerebellum he has to open at the backpart of the head while in an astrocytoma of the frontal area he has to open up the frontpart of the head. I think that perhaps we are giving less credit to the neurosurgeon than he deserves. The neurosurgeon after all is an individual with training, skill and judgement. I don't think he is quite as poorly informed as you suggest.

Dr. Rubinstein: I had the impression that one of the reasons of a system of grading was an attempt to help the neurosurgeon in his work, to assume that he knows nothing about the work of Bailey and Cushing, that he just could not find his way among the maze of histogenetic classification. And as Dr. Netsky pointed out quite rightly the classification was originally put forward by the practical neurosurgeon. That is why it has survived.

Dr. Sayre: Well, the most important change from following the Bailey and Cushing classification to the system of grading is I think that it gets rid of this Cohnheim-Ribbert system. The brain tumours are the same thing as tumours anywhere else in the body. And in my experience in teaching the neurosurgeons if I tell ⸴.em that there is an astrocytoma which is one type of tumour, the glioblastoma multiforme which is another type of tumour, he gets the idea that they are totally different entities. One has to consider that neurosurgeons know something about tumours, while neurologists know nothing about them. It is to give them an idea that these tumours are all members of the same family and they all have similar biological structures.

Dr. Rubinstein: You mean that the idea of the classification was for the benefit of neurologists rather than neurosurgeons?

Dr. Sayre: Pathologist, neurologist, neurosurgeons. Perhaps the greatest value is to the independant general pathologist who is in a hospital where there is now a neurosurgeon. He certainly has to deal with diagnosis of brain tumours and my experience in training general pathologists is that they keep away from all diseases of the brain, because they feel they are so complicated. They are familiar with the system of grading as far as the carcinoma of the breast is concerned or the cancer of the cervix and they can recognize differences in degree of dedifferentiation, anaplasia or whatever term you wish. If they would use these same criteria as far as brain tissue is concerned then they are in a much safer position to give more information as to what type of tumour they are dealing with than if they have to learn that there is an entity called astrocytoma, another called spongioblastoma and another called glioblastoma multiforme.

Dr. Zülch: I still want to ask Dr. Sayre one question about the localisation of the tumours. The localisation or the site of the tumour is really important and I think Dr. Ringertz was already referring to this when he figured out the survival time, because it is no use giving figures like 63 months average survival time if you base yourself on all samples of astrocytoma. Actually the most you can do is compare for instance the astrocytomas of the frontal lobe. You should really only compare the various types of astrocytomas of the frontal lobe, but even there there are fundamental and vital differences. I have been trying to figure out whether there are actual predilection sites for all the gliomas or at least most of the gliomas. For instance there are completely different growth types: if we consider the frontal astrocytomas, the frontomedial type usually has a huge extension into the septum pellucidum. The frontolateral type usually has an extension into the insula and the frontodorsal type has a huge ballooning cyst in the front of the anterior horn. Out of these the frontodorsal type is the most benign; histologically all three are very similar, but one is ballooning out the septum and the other infiltrating down the brain stem, there is then a great difference even in the benign and histologically uniform frontal tumours with regard to survival time. Now if you take into account all the astrocytomas, and I think, you mentioned this example several times, then you get into difficulties, because actually this is not a correct procedure. All it gives you is an overall picture which is approximatively correct, as were the first figures given by Bailey and Cushing where astrocytomas had a 63 months average survival. But the second thing, which seems to me very important from this point of view, is the question whether there are grades 1 to 4 in any location and in any type of tumour: for instance take the ependymoma of the 4th ventricle. Has the ependymoma of the 4th ventricle really several grades of malignancy? Have the ependymomas of the lateral ventricle near the foramen of Monroe several degrees of malignancy at all? And, this is the next question, which makes the whole thing even more puzzling, are the histological differences of these ependymomas in various types really not so great that you cannot compare them? Thus I tried to compare the description of the various types of ependymomas and we found that for instance the ependymoma of the lateral ventricle was a type of its own. It has always the same peculiar appearance. The most curious type we found only in the cerebellopontine angle and the identical picture in the Mayo-paper, I think, comes from there too. So that particular type of ependymoma, whatever you may grade it occurs only in one location of the brain. The spinal cord ependymomas may have a similar architecture, but the above mentioned type which looks almost like a papilloma of the plexus we found only there. The next type will be the most malignant of the ependymomas but of classical architecture, which we find outside the cerebral ventricle, the so-called cerebral ependymomas of youth and they are the most malignant out of the whole group of ependymomas because, even after "total" extirpation very often you have a recurrence after 2, 3 or 4 years, whereas in the case of the ependymoma of the 4th ventricle we have some cases where the surgeon has only split the vermis and the patient has survived 10, 20, even 30 years so that without radical intervention the tumours seem to "dry up". So these observations on the ependymomas make the whole question of grading for me very difficult, because if I adopt the pictures you have given as indicators for the various grades for this class, I would find examples which show that your grade 1 ependymoma is only present in one location, whereas in other locations with equally benign ependymomas I don't find that grade at all. This difficulty in grading and the correlation to prognosis is particularly well shown in the ependymomas. Would you comment on this, Dr. Sayre?

Dr. Sayre: Certainly the histological appearance of ependymomas is quite different, the three sets of varieties grouped originally as the epithelial and papillary variety, the appearance of each is quite different. But they all have about the same prognosis. Originally, when Kernohan brought out his first description of ependymomas, they were in the spinal cord where he found three different histological appearances with these significances. When we talk about grade 2 ependymomas we are discussing ependymomas in which the cellular characteristics, the individual type of cells, the size of the nucleus, the alteration and irregularity of various nuclei are remarkably different. The presence or absence of mitotic figures is extremely variable. These variations are recognized as far as the gross histological appearances is concerned, they are variable, but the cell type is really what the grading is based on, not the way in which the ependymoma forms canals or papillary structures or cell masses. These are all similar in different grades and I have not found them as significant. As far as the differences in tumours in different locations is concerned, Dr. Zülch started the discussion on the frontal lobe and so forth. It is obvious that a tumour which is in the frontal lobe will have a better prognosis than, let's say, a tumour in the parietal lobe which rapidly grows into the internal capsules and gets the parietal fibres. We recently had a patient who had a subtotal removal of an astrocytoma grade 3, of the right frontal lobe. After operation she went back to her work as a beautician and worked for 3 years. Two month before her death she came back because she complained of headache. We were unable to find anything specific about it and sent her home. We heard from her very suddenly when her husband brought her down again because she had had a kind of fit and within about two days there was evidence of increased intracranial pressure and in about 10 days she was dead. This tumour had recurred

not only in the frontal lobe but involved the opposite hemisphere and had
extended down through the internal capsule to the pons. This tumour had
spread tremendously because it had not involved important structures and had
infiltrated between the axis cylinders and thus permitted the axis cylinders to
continue to function. She had continued in her position as a beautician throughout these years with this tumour. Certainly location does make a tremendous
difference and the fact that the surgeon had removed a great portion of the
frontal lobe at the initial operation gave a tremendous space in which it could
grow before it produced the increased intracranial pressure which really was
the actual cause of her death. I believe that location is extremely important,
but I don't believe that I can tell, as a pathologist looking under the microscope,
that this tumour is different or is going to act differently or anything else. This
I think is the problem of the surgeon.

Dr. Zülch: Yes, I only wanted to stress the fact that it is so difficult to get
survival times which are adequate. If you for instance would take the spongioblastoma polare, in Bailey's definition, of the hypothalamus, what would be your
biological prognosis for this group of spongioblastoma? It would be hopeless.
If you take, as I think, the cerebellar "spongioblastic" tumour, the so-called
cerebellar astrocytoma of Bergstrand which I believe is also spongioblastoma.
There, then the spongioblastoma prognosis will be excellent, you see the real
value of overall general figures of survival I remind you of the example, which
we often cited, of the small astrocytoma of the aqueduct which used to kill a
patient in a short time before Torkildsen's procedure was described. Now it gets
a tube in it and survives another 10 years; what then is the genuine prognosis
of such an astrocytoma and how do you get the adequate survival time for
this type?

Dr. Sayre: Bailey's classification has given rise to a problem to be solved
with the use of mass numbers and this is what we have attempt do to. It is a
pleasure for me to see that Dr. Ringertz's figures and my figures are so similar.

Dr. Zülch: May I at the end make a suggestion that we discuss the possibility
of preserving grading on the one hand by combining it with the Bailey/Cushing
classification modified by Penfield at a later occasion. We are all aware of the
need of the neurosurgeon to have a better concept of malignancy than the names
of the Bailey/Cushing classification would be able to give up to now. But this
means to have degrees of malignancy comparable in all brain tumours, I would
suggest to introduce 5 degrees of grading, 0 and 1 to 4 and then to apply these
five grades not to every group but to group all the brain tumours according to
their biological behavior into these five groups.

Perhaps I could give a few more remarks on this type of classification just
at this moment.

Grading of Malignancy of Brain Tumours*

By

K. J. Zülch

Bailey and *Cushing* were the first to estimate the malignancy of tumours on the basis of their extensive clinical experience. This was for the clinician a first and very fruitful advance. They had to take into consideration that in addition to the malignancy of growth there was also a clinical malignancy which in brain tumours more obviously than in any other tumours can differ from malignancy of growth. The other body cavities are elastic so that the results of occupation of space may often remain for a long time

Proposed Scale of Malignancy of Intracranial Tumours According to their Natural Growth

Grade 0	Neurinomas, Meningiomas, Craniopharyngiomas, Pituitary Adenomas, Epidermoids, Dermoids, Teratomas, Lipomas
Grade I	Spongioblastomas, Ependymomas of the Ventricles, Angioblastomas, Plexuspapillomas, Temporo-basal Gangliocytomas
Grade II	Oligodendrogliomas, Astrocytomas, other kinds of Gangliocytomas, Cerebral Ependymomas
Grade III	Pinealomas, Malignant Oligodendrogliomas, Malignant Astrocytomas, Malignant Gangliocytomas, Malignant Meningiomas
Grade IV	Medulloblastomas (Retinoblastomas), Glioblastomas, Primary Sarcomas

scarcely detectable. The situation is quite different with brain tumours where so benign a tumour as the meningioma can be fatal simply as a result of its expansion.

One can only overcome these complications by taking into account the position of a tumour as well as its histological appearances. An astrocytoma of the aqueduct therefore very early becomes a "clinically" malignant tumour while an astrocytoma of the frontal lobe can attain a large size before life becomes threatened.

---

* *Zülch, K. J.,* Die "Gradeinteilung" (Grading) der Malignität der Hirngeschwülste. Acta neurochir., Wien, X (1962), 639—645.

Then as now the clinician was eager to have a complete grading of malignancy and this gave rise to *Broder's* system which provided for 4 grades of malignancy. A similar series of grades was put forward for the uterine cervix. It must of course be recognised that not all carcinomas fall evenly into 4 stages, as for example the carcinomas of the lip which are malignant and fall principally into group 3 and 4 while carcinomas of the rectum which are more benign fall predominantly into grades 1 and 2. Dr. *Sayre* has referred to this in his work. It was with these grading systems in mind that *Kernohan* attempted to devise groups which would reflect the obvious differences in malignancy in various astrocytomas and oligodendrogliomas. He has produced his system of grading in 4 stages which is well known to you and of which we have heard the details from Dr. *Sayre*. Dr. *Ringertz* later sought to simplify this system and only — as is the usual practice in general pathology — used three grades which in regard to the astrocytoma comprised the normal astrocytoma, the intermediate type and the glioblastoma. I have myself attempted a compromise between the grouping of *Bailey* and *Cushing* and the grading system.

My experience has shown me that these 4 grades of malignancy cannot really be applied to all the tumour groups. I have for example endeavoured to establish the characteristic features of the ependymoma and became aware that the ependymoma could vary topographically but that these differences were not simultaneously accompanied by differences in the malignancy of their growth. I also do not believe, that we can distinguish morphologically and biologically 4 different types of oligodendroglioma. One last point is whether one should regard the glioblastoma as the malignant form of the astrocytoma. There certainly do occur glioblastomas which have developed secondarily from astrocytomas as *Scherer* has shown but the majority have obviously developed as primary malignant tumours.

So I am not convinced that we should divide each tumour group into 4 grades. On the other hand there are definite differences in malignancy between the astrocytoma and the astrocytoma which has undergone malignant change, the oligodendroglioma and the oligodendroglioma which has undergone malignancy. In a similar manner the ependymoma of the cerebral hemispheres in the younger age groups with its numerous mitoses is semi-malignant while the remaining ependymomas belong to the benign tumours. In a grading system the extracerebral tumours should be accorded a position indicating their greater benignity.

How is one to achieve such a system which will take into account at the same time the experiences of the *Bailey-Cushing* group and that of the *Kernoham* group? I believe *Hamperl* has in the literature made the suggestion for the first time, simply out of practical experience: that there should be a system with 5 grades of malignancy designated 0 to 4 and an attempt made to place all recognized tumour groups in this system, so that one would not end up with 5 malignant grades different in each group which cannot be compared with one another. Such a system I will now project on the wall. We will leave it there so that you can take in the details. I would place the purely space-occupying tumours as for example the meningiomas, neurinomas, craniopharyngiomas and pituitary tumours in group 0 and in group 1 the intracerebral tumours of benign nature such as the spongioblastoma, angioblastoma, ependymoma of the ventricles and papilloma of the choroid plexus. In the second group we can place the normal astrocytoma and oligodendroglioma as well as the cerebral ependymoma of the younger age group. In most of these cases one may anticipate a survival period of 3 to 5 years. In group 3 come the malignant forms of oligodendroglioma and astrocytoma; and in group 4 we finally place the absolutely malignant sympathico- and retino-blastoma, medulloblastoma, glioblastoma and the sarcomas. We would this way, I believe, achieve a very balanced tumour classification of malignancy for which the surgeon who is very appreciative of a plastic demonstration of malignancy would be most grateful.

Discussion

Dr. Zülch: Dr. Sayre, would you comment on a compromise like this?

Dr. Sayre: I believe this is quite helpful. I do not object to the term grading being applied to this particular classification, but, unfortunately, as grading has been used with different connotation, if the same word is used it would lead to confusion. Grouping or some other term separate from grading might be better. Certainly otherwise it has many merits.

Dr. Rubinstein: I want to add that in actual practice the grading classification of the Mayo clinic and Dr. Ringertz is widely adopted, particularly in the United States, also in many parts of England and in Scandinavia. I don't think that this grouping in any way replaces it. It is to the credit of the classification of the Mayo Clinic that many pathologists have a fairly good concept of what grade 1, 2, 3 or 4 astrocytoma.

Dr. Zülch: Yes, but you have seen that quite a good many members of this group who have some experience in the tumour classification have very strong objections against it. My suggestion aims at giving meaningful comparison of the various tumour groups. I think this would give the neurosurgeons who are used to a classification according to Bailey/Cushing a good idea where a particular tumour stands in relation to various other groups. But we have not heard a word yet from you, Dr. Kersting, about grading from the point of view of your experiences with tissue culture. Are there any comments to be made?

Dr. Kersting: There is no definite comment to be made. I know that Dr. Lumsden finds the system of grading of the Kernohan school can be adapted to the tissue culture conditions. We could not confirm that so far and neither could a group of Hungarian workers on tissue culture.

Dr. Woolf: I would like to say that in this discussion on grading systems we heard about the value of grading for neurosurgeons and even neurologists, but there are other people who are concerned with patients with cerebral tumours the general physicians and even the general practitioners, and I would imagine this last system could be very valuable to them, but only if it were co-ordinated with grading of tumours throughout the rest of the body, so when a general practitioner or a general physician gets a report from the surgeon operating — let's say with the pathologist's report saying that this is a grade 2 tumour he should know that it has about the same malignancy as certain renal tumours, I wonder whether the opinion of Dr. Hamperl could be heard on this and, whether there might be a possibility of extending this system of grading to enable comparisons to be made with extracranial tumours.

Dr. Zülch: Could you, Dr. Ringertz, as a general pathologist, help us?

Dr. Ringertz: I think that this may be of some help because experience comes to the pathologist working with neurosurgeons as to what in different brain tumours are the rate of growth and the outcome in respect of the survival of the patient on the whole. But there are naturally difficulties because in some cases you have taken location into account and in other cases you have neglected location.

Dr. Zülch: Well, I have taken it into account only if for example the epen-dymomas located outside the cerebral ventricles have a completely different behavior from other ependymomas. You see, this group of extraventricular cerebral ependymomas in youth, which we have studied very carefully in the last twenty years, definitely has a poor prognosis.

Dr. Ringertz: Yes, it has a poorer prognosis. Moreover, I would like to have in group 3 with malignant oligodendroglioma, also malignant ependymoma. I don't think this scheme can actually be put instead of the grading of the Mayo Clinic but it would help to put it as an appendix to the classification list just to give the surgeons the opinion of the pathologist as to the general behavior of the tumours. So I think it is very worth to think over this system.

Dr. Zülch: This could be the object of another meeting of this group and if there are no comments in the moment, I think we close this session. Thank you.

III. Spongioblastoma

Chairman: I open the session on the definition of the spongioblastomas of the brain.

Some Remarks on the Spongioblastoma of the Brain*

By

K. J. Zülch

Bailey and *Cushing* introduced the name spongioblastoma unipolare in their system after the term had already been used for other tumours, probably for the first time by *Kaufmann* and later by *Ribbert,* in connection with an ependymoma-like tumour. The term "spongioblastoma unipolare" was not altogether satisfactory since the type of glioma to which *Bailey* and *Cushing* applied it consisted largely of bipolar cells. They sought however to make a distinction between this tumour and the spongioblastoma multiforme, a term which *Globus* and *Strauss* had in the meantime made popular. *Bailey* and *Cushing* pointed out that the spongioblasts were well demonstrated with gold sublimate in the spongioblastoma unipolare in which there were many immature astrocytes. The tumour had a predilection for the cerebellum and the chiasma and IIIrd ventricle. The average survival period was very long most of the tumours growing slowly in spite of the unfavourable location in many cases.

In spite of this description of the spongioblastoma in the cerebellum, it is obvious that the majority of these tumours in the literature have been described as astrocytomas. This was later criticized by *Bergstrand* of whom I shall speak later.

At present I will only mention that *Penfield* has placed the spongioblastoma in the group of poorly defined gliomas, at the same time pointing out that they occur predominantly in early life and usually in the cerebellum. He refers to the striking discrepancy between the position of the unipolar spongioblastoma in the glioma system — it should according to its position consist predominantly of immature cells — and its relatively long survival period. However he also is prepared to accept the majority of polar spongioblastomas of the cerebellum and cerebral hemispheres as piloid

* *Zülch, K. J.,* Das Glioblastom, morphologisch und biologisch gesehen. Acta neurochir., Wien, Suppl. *VI* (1959), 1—30. — *Zülch, K. J.,* and *A. Nover,* Die Spongioblastome des Sehnerven. Graefes Arch. Ophth. *161* (1960), 405—419.

astrocytomas. The first discussion of this tumour group at a meeting of the Association of British Neurosurgeons in 1937 in Berlin was opened by *Bergstrand*. He reported 10 benign cystic tumours of the cerebellar vermis which could not on histological evidence be accepted as astrocytomas. They obviously did not correspond histologically with the astrocytoma described by *Bailey* and *Cushing* not at any rate as it occurs in the cerebral hemispheres. The majority of the cells are made up of unipolar and bipolar spongioblasts which most closely resemble the embryonic glia. Particularly characteristic are the corkscrew-like processes which can ultimately resemble the end of a whip-lash. The majority of the cells are derived from astrocytes, so that one encounters a mixture of spongioblasts, ill-defined embryonic cells and astrocytes, i. e. the various developmental stages of the glia. His later work on the cerebellar astrocytoma has certainly somewhat weakened this excellent report, but I do not wish to discuss it further now. At the same time of *Bergstrand's* criticisms, *Zülch* for the first time pointed out the occurence of numerous *Rosenthal* fibres in these tumours. He mentioned a few classical descriptions in the early literature in which this type of tumour was particularly well recognized.

Zülch completely agreed with *Bergstrand's* criticism and was of the opinion that the majority of these so-called astrocytomas of the cerebellum corresponded with the spongioblastoma of the cerebellum of *Bailey*. Certainly there are still some discrepances because in *Cushing's* book a few of the tumours in this same group were classified as fibrillary astrocytomas and others as spongioblastomas in a similar way to *Penfield*. There are in the literature large treatises in particular those of *Bucy* and *Gustavson* and of *Ringertz* and *Nordenstam*, which give practically an identical account to those of *Bailey* and *Cushing, Zülch* and *Bergstrand* which *correspond* to the original description by *Bailey* and *Eisenhardt*.

Zülch has often referred in his later work to this tumour group and expressed the opinion that we are dealing here with a tumour of the subependymal glia in the form described in detail by *Opalski*, i. e. a mixture of different types of cells ranging from mature astro- cytes to spindle cells corresponding to spongioblasts. One also finds in chronic inflammation a tissue which is very similar to that of the tumour. In individual places there are *Rosenthal* fibres by which — again as a single tumour group — the polar spongioblastoma — in *Bailey's* sense — is characterized.

Dorothy Russell and *Russell* and *Rubinstein* have defined the spongioblastoma in a different way. They rightly point out that if th ᵥ spongioblastoma is to be cytologically representative of the migrating spongioblast it must be composed of very delicate, slender, short cells with scanty neuroglial fibrils. Biologically it should grow rapidly and be malignant. Such tumours have been seen and described by these authors and are distinguished by them quite justifiably from the spongioblastoma polare as defined by *Bailey* and the other authors.

Dr. *Rubinstein* has kindly allowed us to see his sections, and I would like to suggest that we are dealing here with a special type of tumour which is certainly extremely uncommon. I have only once seen a similar tumour in the cerebral hemispheres (described in 1940) which I left unclassified, but regarded as a transitional form between spongioblastoma and ependymoma. I would put forward a similar interpretation for *Russell* and *Rubinstein's* tumour. This grows predominantly in the IVth ventricle, but is definitely infiltrating at its borders. We shall be able by projection to have an opportunity to acquaint ourselves more completely with this tumour.

Kersting has recently reported on the culture of a series of spongioblastomas, although up to the present only cerebellar astrocytomas have been successfully cultured. He found long bipolar cells with long fine protoplasmic processes. In some areas a few spongioblasts gathered together in streams and bundles. They were very similar in the late stage to the cell type of the cerebellar astrocytoma. In this stage there also occurred a few small multipolar astrocytes, which were however in a very small minority as compared with the bipolar cells.

I now come to the finer structure of the polar spongioblastoma according to *Bailey's* definition, but first I would like to make clear the two main problems. The first concerns the definition and delineation of this tumour, which one believes to be a single entity. Not only does the histological picture — here we must agree with *Bergstrand* — allow the spongioblastoma to be distinguished from the cerebral astrocytoma but the survival period is clearly much longer than is typical of the cerebral astrocytoma, and this in spite of the particularly unfavourable localisation of the spongioblastoma. We must in addition concern ourselves with the naming of the tumour and this may be one of the most difficult points in the discussion on the polar spongioblastoma.

In a discussion with our Spanish friends in 1955 * we agreed on the vague and certainly far too neutral name of polar glioma as a

---

* *Obrador Alcalde, S., K. J. Zülch,* and *J. S. Ibanez,* Discusion from: Rev. españ. oncol. *IV* (1955), 163—171.

working hypothesis. *Zülch* has discussed whether one might not use the terms subependymoma or ependymal glioma for this purpose. Both of these were etymologically acceptable but unfortunately had been used for other tumours. Perhaps one should therefore allow a little time for discussion of a suitable name.

I will now quickly run through with you the biological and morphological characteristics of the spongioblastoma as defined by us.

The spongioblastoma is predominantly a tumour of youth, the female sex is more commonly affected, it occurs in various sites but always near the ventricles for example in the ventricular wall, in the chiasma, in the hypothalamus, in the midbrain, pons, IVth ventricle, aqueduct, cerebellar vermis and optic tract, in the neigbourhood of the old optic vesicle and finally in the midline of the spinal cord. Histologically it is a tumour of average cellularity with spindle cells predominating with oval nuclei which are mostly arranged in long streams and without any increase in mitoses. There is plentiful formation of glial fibres which can be recognized with metal impregnation very easily and which *Bergstrand* has shown particularly well. The tumour infiltrates the cerebral tissue and grows into the leptomeninges which it widely separates. The spongioblastoma has a tendency to liquefaction and in particular to the formation of little cysts. In many places the tissue resembles that of an oligodendroglioma as has been mentioned earlier. Normally the tumour has only a few vessels which are mostly capillaries, but it may in places show a great richness in vessels which suggests that a dysembryogenetic character already existed at the time of the ingrowth of the mesenchyme. Such angiogliotic "mixed tumours" have been many times described in the literature and we have ourselves presented a similar tumour of the cerebral hemisphere in the Cancer-Symposium in Denver/Colorado in 1957 *.

There are of course also secondary vascular formations, particularly in the form of vascular loops and glomeruli which one has for a long time, though incorrectly, regarded as characteristic of the glioblastoma multiforme. They are in fact much more common in all benign tumours and occur even in the neurinomas.

Calcification occurs in the form of small deposits of calcium. Sometimes individual vessels are calcified. Only occasionally does the spongioblastoma show calcification radiographically. In 1940 we reported three such heavily calcified cerebellar astrocytomas of which one has been reported by *Bergstrand*.

---

* Cancer Seminar Vol. II, No. 3 (1957).

And now in conclusion we may refer to two very interesting peculiarities of this tumour group. Firstly the already mentioned formation of *Rosenthal* fibres, which in recent years have attracted several scientific and particularly histochemical investigations From these we can now say that the fibres are not related to haemoglobin breakdown products but that the earlier concepts which I myself have advocated — that they are degeneration products of the glial fibre — are probably valid. Related to them is a second very peculiar structure which takes the form of "granular bodies" occuring in very many of these cases. Here one is obviously again dealing with a degeneration of the cells with different histochemical peculiarities, as *Diezel* has shown. But its presence can be accepted as positive evidence of a spongioblastoma *. Up to now we have not seen them in any other tumour.

The cases which our friend Dr. *Calvo* has provided for examination for this symposium, one of which was sited in the cerebellum and the other two in the chiasma are also in agreement with this description.

Now perhaps we could hear first from Dr. *Rubinstein* because he represents the opposing view and then we would be most grateful if the participants from the different special fields would tell us what has been discovered in these fields in regard to the spongioblastoma. Thus Dr. *Luginbühl* should tell us what happens in animals, Dr. *Müller* can speak to us on the histochemical reactions, while Dr. *Woolf* could speak to us about the electron microscopic findings. Dr. *Netsky* and Dr. *Schiefer* may tell us whether it has been possible to produce tumours experimentally and how they behave with transplantation. I hope that in this way we may have a lively discussion on this group which should centre around two points:

1. Whether there is a tumour entity clearly separable from the cerebellar astrocytoma and which *Bailey* in support of this contention has designated as polar spongioblastoma but which many authors have classified as cerebellar astrocytoma and
2. what name should we now give to this group.

Discussion

Dr. *Zülch:* Before we go into the discussion of this I would like to get a more precise concept of Prof. Dorothy Russell and Dr. Rubinstein's views on the spongioblastomas. We call upon you, Dr. Rubinstein.

---

* *Diezel, P. B.,* und *E. Rottmann,* Histochemische Untersuchungen an Rosenthalschen Fasern in Ependymgranulationen und im Spongioblastom. Dtsch. Zschr. Nervenhk. *177* (1958), 222—234.

Discussion on Polar Spongioblastomas

By

L. J. Rubinstein

With 5 Figures

The problem of the so-called "polar spongioblastoma" of *Bailey* [1] and a historical review of this controversial group have been clearly outlined by Dr. *Zülch* in his report.

In practice, it is apparent that the label "polar spongioblastoma" is frequently and, in our view, unjustifiably, applied by various authorities to two types of tumor, widely different in their histological and biological characters, though both tend to be midline in location and to occur in children and young subjects.

First, the fairly common pontine glioma, which constitutes the well-recognized "diffuse hypertrophy" of older authors, and in which the pons is diffusely replaced by an extensive, ill-defined neoplastic process. Histologically and biologically, these tumors have many features which link them to the diffuse cerebral astro·cytomas of adults. They are usually composed of elongated, bipolar cells; in common with astrocytomas which infiltrate the corpus callosum and the internal capsule, these appearance are almost certainly to be ascribed to a diffuse penetration of the neoplastic cells along pre-existing nerve-fibre tracts, therefore constituting a variety of "secondary structures" within the terms of *Scherer's* definition [8]. Thus, the polar cells of the tumor tend to occupy the more basal portion of the pons, whereas the tegmental areas usually contain stellate astrocytes. Furthermore, as in the diffuse cerebral astrocytomas of adults, there is the same tendency to undergo anaplasia, especially in the central part of the growth, resulting in a histological picture indistinguishable from that of glioblastoma multiforme; an event we have demonstrated in sixty per cent of the examples in our material. It seems therefore unjustifiable in our view to regard these tumors as other than diffuse astrocytomas which frequently progress to a malignant phase.

The second group constitutes an entirely different variety of glioma. There is, to be sure, no difficulty in agreeing on the identity of the neoplasm we are all dealing with, and our observations would tend to support the separation of this group into a relatively circumscribed and histologically benign tumor with a predominance-though not an exclusive one-for the optic nerves and chiasm, the hypothalamus, and the wall of the third ventricle. It occurs mainly-though again not exclusively-in children and young subjects. The microscopic features are quite distinctive. The tumor cells are mostly elongated, thin and tapering. They are often arranged in parallel formations and characteristically ensheath the blood vessels longitudinally. Stout neuroglial fibrils are easily demonstrated, and many areas are prone to undergo microcystic degeneration. But in such areas the preserved cells are not piloid but feebly stellate, and many of these appear to be protoplasmic astrocytes. The characteristic degenerative changes referred to in the literature as "cytoid bodies" or "Rosenthal fibers" are often found in this group. We have also gained the impression that there is a definite kinship, both biological and histological, between these tumors and the cerebellar astrocytomas. Because of their relatively benign character, and since the component cells recall the appearances of reactive astrocytes of piloid form, we have included these tumors amongst the general group of the astrocytomas and, following *Penfield* [3], labelled them "piloid or pilocytic". In an attempt, however, to separate them from their more diffuse and more malignant couterparts which infiltrate the cerebrum and brainstem, we have recently suggested, that the term "piloid astrocytoma of juvenile type" might conveniently designate them [7].

The reasons why the name "polar spongioblastoma" seems inappropriate to this entity are therefore prompted by the following considerations:

1. Biologically, these tumors are, by common consent, relatively benign and slowly-growing. The term "spongioblastoma" implies a primitive tumor of high malignancy.

2. Histologically, the elongated glial cells are, we believe, differentiated astrocytes, usually bipolar, and showing many coarse, well-defined neuroglial cytoplasmic fibrils, unlike the embryonic cells generally understood as "spongioblasts".

3. Though many polar cells are present, these tumors also contain large numbers of stellate astrocytes, often best visualized in those areas which show early degenerative changes.

4. Tissue culture of two of these tumors-one from the hypothalamic region, the other from the cerebellum-undertaken by *Russell* and *Bland* [5] in 1934, demonstrated that the migrated cells had the typical morphology of astrocytes. The more recent work of *Lumsden* [2] supports this interpretation.

5. Several points of similarity with the cerebellar astrocytomas are acknowledged. Though, in many cases, the latter have a distinctive histological pattern, some examples are indistinguishable from the juvenile type of piloid astrocytoma as encountered in the region of the third ventricle or, very occasionally, in the cerebral hemispheres. In the cerebellar tumors, it is, however, possible that the pilocytic features might be ascribed to an origin from the Bergmann glia, which are normally polar. At all events, the labelling, as it has been suggested [9], of all cerebellar astrocytomas as "spongioblasto-

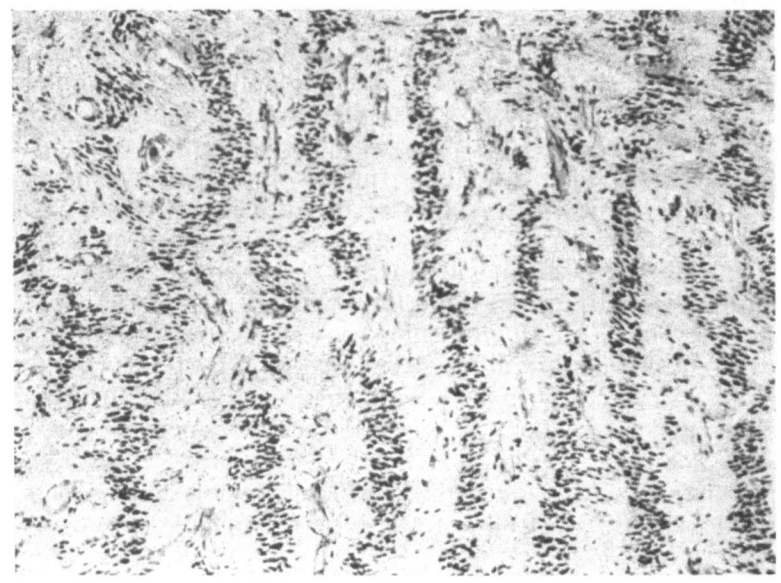

Fig. 1. Polar spongioblastoma. Case 2 of Russell and Cairns (1947). Typical arrangement of tumor cells in palisades. Silver carbonate (triple) method 95 ×.

mas" would lead to a paradoxical situation in which, in any general classification of the astrocytomas, those arising in the cerebellum, as well as in the optic nerve and the spinal cord, would have to be specifically excluded, notwithstanding the normal presence of astrocytes in these regions. This position is, we feel, hard to defend.

6. Finally, there arises the question whether true polar spongioblastomas exist as a separate entity. In 1947, *Russell* and *Cairns* [6] reported four cases of glioma in children and adolescents which, though rare, possess an individuality which renders them easily recognizable at first glance under the microscope. The tumors were closely related to the ventricular system and cerebrospinal metastases were confirmed histologically in two cases. There was no

doubt as to the biological malignancy of these neoplasms. Histologically, the majority of the component cells had the primitive morphological features which recalled the spongioblasts as seen in histological preparations of the fetal cerebrum of 10 and 18 weeks, and these authors felt that the term "polar spongioblastoma" was the appropriate one for this tumor, a view reiterated by *Dorothy Russell* [4] in 1955, when she drew attention to its possible kinship with some forms of medulloblastoma.

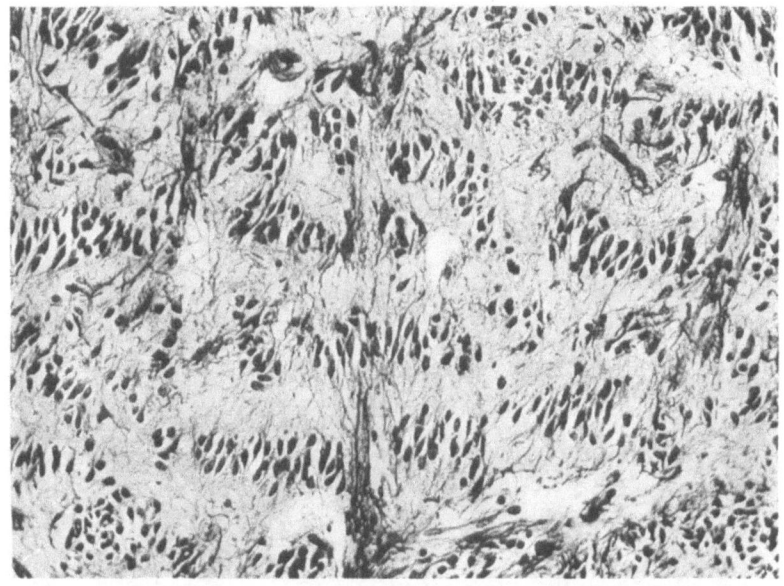

Fig. 2. Polar spongioblastoma. Case 3 of Russell and Cairns (1947). Typical palisade arrangement of finely fibrillated polar cells. Mallory's P. T. A. H. 220 ×.

Figs. 1 to 5 illustrate the distinctive morphological features of two of the cases originally described by *Russell* and *Cairns* [6]. Fig. 1 demonstrates the architecture of a central brainstem tumor in a male of 16 (case 2), where bundles of thin parallel uni- and bipolar cells are arranged so as to produce a remarkable palisade effect, the pattern being quite regular throughout the tissue. A similar arrangement is present in another example (case 3), from a fourth ventricle tumor in a two and a half year-old boy, with leptomeningeal metastases over the lumbar enlargement and cauda equina: the fine fibrillation of the polar cells, and their delicate cytoplasmic processes are demonstrated in both P. T. A. H. preparations (Fig. 2) and by the silver carbonate method (Fig. 3). As shown

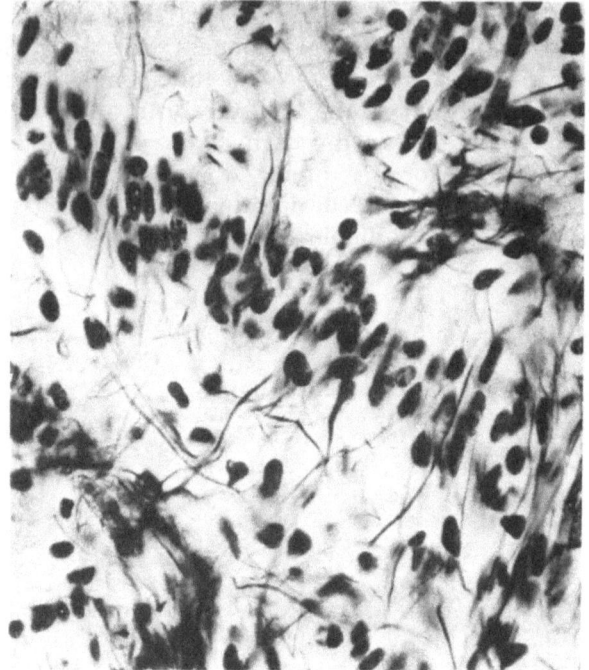

Fig. 3.

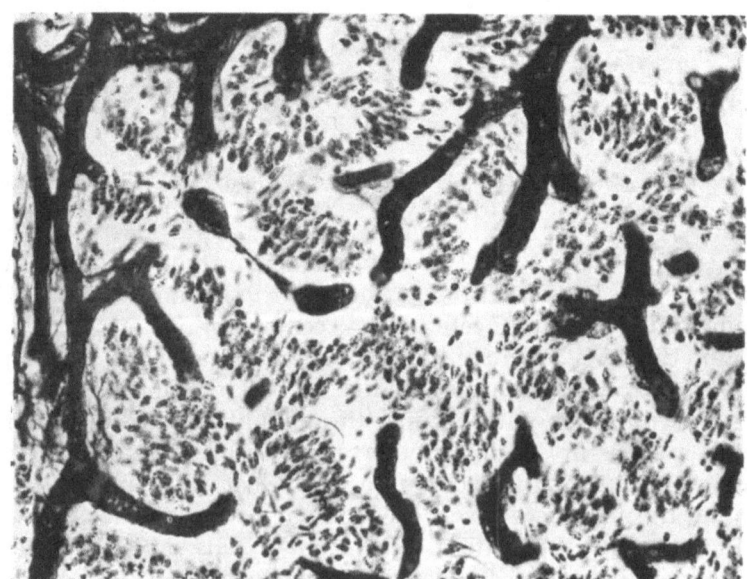

Fig. 4.

in Fig. 4, a connective-tissue stain emphasizes the grouping of the tumor cells in compact masses separated and supported by an anastomosing network of collagenous and vascular trabeculae. In a few areas, the neuroglial fibers were stained more strongly and coarser in appearance; here a variable number of stellate cells are seen, interpreted as relatively immature astrocytes and indicative of an early differentiation of the spongioblastic element (Fig. 5). A similar mixture of both the more and less differentiated cells was noted in the spinal metastases of this case.

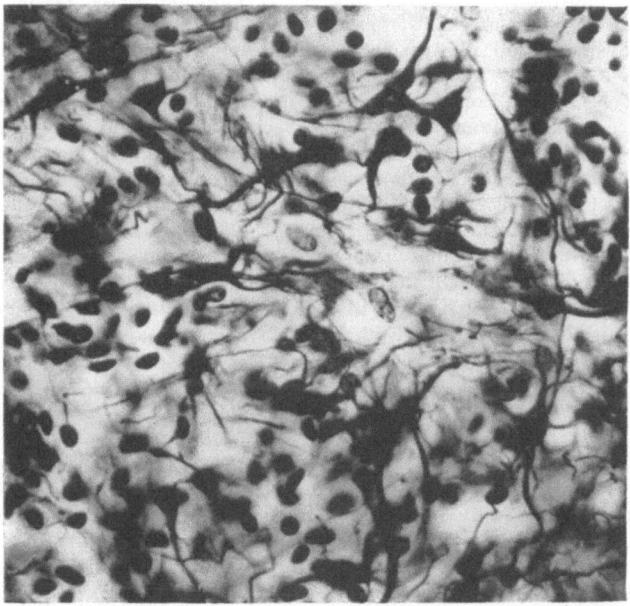

Fig. 5. Same case as Fig. 2. Focus of small stellate cells (immature astrocytes), representing differentiation in a polar spongioblastoma. Silver carbonate method 450 ×.

Biologically and histologically, these tumors are therefore quite distinct from the piloid astocytomas of juvenile type. They are extremely rare. Since the four original cases reported by *Russell* and *Cairns,* we have in recent years seen only two further examples of this kind from outside collections, one of which will be briefly referred to in the subsequent discussions of this Symposium, in

Fig. 3. Same case as Fig. 2. Delicate cytoplasmic processes and fibrils of unipolar cells, impregnated with silver. Silver carbonate method 530 ×.

Fig. 4. Same case as Fig. 2. Arrangement of tumor cells in compact masses separated by an anastomosing vascular connective-tissue stroma. Silver carbonate method for reticulin 200 ×.

relation to the mixed gliomas. However, since both the age incidence and their location coincide with those of the relatively frequent piloid astrocytoma of juvenile type, it is likely that, in any large series of so-called "spongioblastomas", there may be a small number of examples which, if recognized, might fall within the category of what we believe to be true polar spongioblastoma. The further recording of such cases seems highly desirable.

References

1. *Bailey, P.,* and *L. Eisenhardt,* Spongioblastomas of the Brain. J. Comp. Neurol., Philadelphia, *56* (1932), 391. — 2. *Lumsden, C. E.,* Tissue Culture in Relation to Tumours of the Nervous System. In: Pathology of Tumours of the Nervous System, by D. S. Russell, and L. J. Rubinstein. Edw. Arnold, London, 1959. — 3. *Penfield, W.,* Cytology and Cellular Pathology of the Nervous System. Vol. 2. Hoeber. New York, 1932. — 4. *Russell, D. S.,* Polar Spongioblastomas: Their Place in the Glioma Series. Proc. Second Int. Cong. Neuropath. London, *1* (1955), 259. — 5. *Russell, D. S.,* and *J. O. W. Bland,* Further Notes on the Tissue Culture of Gliomas with Special Reference to Bailey's Spongioblastoma. J. Path. Bact. *39* (1934), 375. — 6. *Russell, D. S.,* and *H. Cairns,* Polar Spongioblastomas. Arch. histol., B. Aires, *3* (1947), 423. — 7. *Russell, D. S.,* and *L. J. Rubinstein,* Pathology of Tumours of the Nervous System. Edw. Arnold, London, 1959. — 8. *Scherer, H. J.,* Structural Development in Gliomas. Amer. J. Cancer *34* (1938), 333. — 9. *Zülch, K. J.,* Biologie und Pathologie der Hirngeschwülste. Handbuch der Neurochirurgie. Edited by H. Olivecrona and W. Tönnis. Springer. Berlin, 1956, vol. 3.

Discussion

Dr. Zülch: Two or three different types of tumours have been labelled already as spongioblastomas in the literature of the last 5 decades. We saw your beautiful preparations last night and I think that nobody will disagree that these were an entity of its own, but a very rare one. Without much discussion we would also — though only theoretically — admit that the name of spongioblastoma is not too bad for this group, but as you know and as Dr. Hamperl said, there is a discrepancy between the theoretical value of a term and the practical acceptance of this term in the world of classification of brain tumours. Before we start, the general discussion perhaps, Dr. Kersting will comment on this?

Dr. Kersting: Well, I have to concentrate entirely on the astrocytoma of juvenile type the so-called cerebellar astrocytoma or spongioblastoma as I have not seen any of the cases you showed in the last part of your paper. Before giving you a short survey of the tissue culture results in this group of tumours I think it is interesting to point out that a "spongioblast" never occurs in tissue cultures of embryonic foetal brain tissue. Thus we accept the spongioblast only in the sense of Paul Weiss as a modulation not as an entity and another point may be of interest regarding the proposal of Dr. Zülch to call them subependymomas. You saw Dr. Zülch's picture of two slides of spinal cord with spongioblastoma around the central canal. Now we have had 6 cases of these during 4 years and they were operated upon. Certainly we did not get all the material but all these tumours were so far quite similar. A large part with a spongioblastic appearance and another large part with an ependymoma-like appearance and we cut from them one half for ordinary histological section and one half for tissue culture explantation, and three of these six showed in tissue culture ependymoma-like structures and the other three showed what we called the spongioblastic appearance. But I am not going to comment further on this because the particles we had to explant were very small. But it would be interesting if this could be confirmed later on. Now as to the cerebellar spongioblastoma we have had about 15 tumours of this sort explanted. There is no difference between or among those tumours, regardless as to whether they are highly degenerated histologically or not, whether they are highly cellular without any cystic degeneration or whether they have cystic degeneration. These features cannot be detected in tissue culture. So the proliferation in our cultures starts with the emergence of bundles of long elongated cells, coming out of the explants. This in within the first 12 hours after explantation. During the next days and weeks a network of very fine spindle cells is formed. This distinguishes the cerebellar astrocytoma or spongioblastoma cerebelli from the fusiform glioblastoma. If we explant a fusiform glioblastoma in a suspension of single cells, then we get a network, but this network is not a "genuine" formation of the tissue but is imposed by the mode of explantation. Thus I emphasize the point that we get a genuine network formed in the spongioblastoma of the cerebellum but not in fusiform glioblastomas, although the structure of single cells, may be very similar. If we start explantation from the beginning with a very diluted medium so that practically no outgrowth appears, then we get after days and days the migration of very small cells. Then you see a few elongated cells although it is still mostly a very small migration of small stellate cells. And the picture of the normal outgrowth i. e. if we have a big proliferation and push it and then stop it and try to make it differentiate into stellate astrocytes — this does not occur with the spongioblastoma cerebelli. This is a difference that distinguishes this sort of tumours definitely from the cerebral astrocytoma which I showed yesterday.

Dr. Rubinstein: May I just ask you one question, Dr. Kersting. The previous slide was taken from a cerebral tumour, or was it cerebellar?

Dr. Kersting: A cerebellar tumour, only with a very diluted medium and we got no real proliferation in other parts of this tumour. The other explantations of this tumour showed exactly the same picture as I showed before. I can't tell you whether the photograph I showed, was of exatly the same tumour.

Dr. Rubinstein: How do you interpret these stellate cells here?

Dr. Kersting: Not yet, I can not yet, you see, I give you first the facts. Well, let us go back to the first question of whether a spongioblast occurs in foetal brain tissue. Foetal brain tissue after about 8 days of cultivation shows differentiation of neuroglia from the primary neuroepithelium. We get in tissue culture when explanting foetal brain tissue, a "neuroepithelium", which means an epithelium-like sheet of neural origin. That has nothing to do with the term neuroepithelium as the embryologist uses it. A larger magnification shows that spongioblasts really do not exist. One may not be sure whether the cells are really astrocytes and perhaps those in the left corner are oligodendrocytes I cannot determine them in every case. One would perhaps call those in the centre astrocytes and some of the others oligodendrocytes. As I said yesterday to Dr. Calvo, it would be extremely helpful to us to have selective stainings with several metallic impregnations adapted to tissue culture conditions, because so far it had not been shown that there is such a selectivity. Thank you very much.

Dr. Rubinstein: These pictures and your findings, Dr. Kersting, were quite remarkable, but I must say that so far as I can see, they would rather tend to support the concept that your so-called cerebellar spongioblastomas are in fact astrocytomas rather than the reverse because you have shown very beautiful small astrocytes. There is no disagreement, I think, between your findings and the original ones of Dorothy Russell as far as I can assess. The second point concerns the mixture of ependymal cells and spongioblasts in the spinal cord. I am not certain whether these tumours do fall into this particular group, because I have seen ependymomas of the spinal cord composed partly of ependymal cells and partly of cells with long polar processes and I am not at all certain that they are anything like the cells we are discussing at the moment.

Dr. Zülch: I entirely agree with the analysis of the tumour cells shown in the tissue cultures. They correspond to what Bergstrand beautifully showed in his first paper *. And he stressed that you can have astrocytes or astrocyte-like cells, but on the other hand you have many elements which are definitely different from the ordinary astrocytes of ordinary cerebral astrocytomas because of all these long screwlike structures in bundles which he compared with the hair of a young girl. And there is the formation of Rosenthal fibres. We have looked for them in cerebral astrocytomas for a long long time, but have never seen them. All these points suggest that this form of astrocytic glia if you like to call it this way is a special glia. Part of the cells then may look like astrocytes, but they are different from the components of the cerebral astrocytoma. That's the point, because if we classify them together with cerebral astrocytoma then a wrong biological labelling will be given. Even if you call them pilocytic astrocytomas, it seems inappropriate, because sometimes if the cerebral astrocytoma grows into the corpus callosum or into some myelin bundles then you get long elongated astrocytes and you can have a beautiful astrocytoma piloideum in the definition of Penfield and Dorothy Russell and yet this is a different tumour from that we are speaking about. It is like a sarcoma growing into the cornea, where you have this type of elongated cell which like red cells push themselves through the little tubular spaces between the myelin sheaths. I think most of us agree on the definition of this group. It is a special group. It contains astrocyte-like cells. The name spongioblastoma is definitely very bad, but how do we get out of this situation; that is the point if we have in mind Dr. Hamperl's rules on terminology. We may agree that biologically and histologically it is different from the cerebral astrocytoma and that on the other hand theoretically or histogenetically speaking Dorothy Russell's type of tumour deserves far more the name of spongioblastoma than the other one.

Dr. Rubinstein: Well, having invoked the polar spongioblast for what we call the true polar spongioblastoma we had to find another name for the Bailey type. And that is why we tried to resolve the problem by adding "juvenile type" to it, because I agree with you that these pilocytic forms are different from the diffuse piloid astrocytoma of the cerebrum. I want to add something about the Rosenthal fibres. We have seen one case which we have illustrated in which Rosenthal fibres were present in a very superficial cerebral astrocytoma of the parietal lobe.

Dr. Ringertz: In a paper I have written about the so-called cerebellar astrocytoma, naturally as Dr. Zülch has already mentioned, I shared the concept

---

* *Bergstrand, H.,* Über das sogenannte Astrocytom des Kleinhirns. Virch. Arch. path. Anat. *287* (1932), 538. — *Bergstrand, H.,* Weiteres über sogenannte Kleinhirnastrocytome. Virch. Arch. path. Anat. *299* (1937), 725—739.

that this tumour is quite different from the cerebral astrocytoma, and I defined it as a polar spongioblastoma which inclines to this formation of special vascular arrangements and of Rosenthal fibres. Naturally also I then became interested as to whether this type of tumour occured in other parts of the brain and I found that they really do occur in typical form in many locations, even in the cerebral hemispheres. In the consecutive material during 10 years I found that 11% of the cerebral hemisphere astrocytomas where in structure similar to the cerebellar astrocytomas. Amongst the central benign gliomas of the pons, of the medulla, the basal nuclei and quadrigeminal region I also foud many tumours which corresponded very closely to the cerebellar type. But in addition there were of course in these locations a majority of gliomas correponding to the ordinary astrocytoma type. But between these different poles I could define an intermediate group which I called polar spongioblastomas not of cerebellar type. I mean that in these tumours you could stain very bipolar spongioblasts but also very many astrocytes, more stellate astrocytes than in the cerebellar type where you also find them but in very much smaller numbers. You could in this intermediate type find Rosenthal fibres, cystic degeneration and glomerulation of the small vessels, but not to the extent seen in the typical cerebellar tumour. So I think that there are perhaps in some regions tumours which are difficult to classify and beween these ordinary astrocytomas and the bipolar spongioblastomas a tumour composed of two components really seems to exist. Now when we come to the suprasellar gliomas you find there also rather characteristic bipolar spongioblasts and also stellate astrocytic elements. In the tumours of the optic tract you have perhaps also a sort of mechanical moulding of the glial structure so that by mechanical compression the impression is given of a piloid arrangement of the glia and I think it is possible that in some of the pontine gliomas this element of mechanical compression between the bundles of myelin fibres is at work. But in my opinion mechanical compression can't account for the fact so many of the cells clearly look like bipolar elements. They could not be bipolar just by compression. The bundles of glia could be parallel through compression but not really the cell body and its processes. Therefore I think that we should have this group of bipolar spongioblastoma. It is not a good name because the term "bipolar" should be rare. To summarize I feel that this group exists not only in the cerebellum, but in the central brain stem and in the suprasellar region and finaly I want to stress that a minority of the hemisphere astrocytomas are of this type, the form exists as a type and they are very circumscribed and their prognosis when operated upon is quite similar to the cerebellar astrocytoma and much better than that of the other cerebral astrocytomas. We have now in the Stockholm material more then 40 of such cases of which 11 seem to have the same structure and the same biology.

Dr. Zülch: Thank you, Dr. Ringertz. I raised this question and I think we need in addition to hear the concept of the Hortega group on the question of optic tumours and spongioblastomas. I would like you, Dr. Calvo, particularly to discuss the concept of Hortega that these tumours in the chiasm were actually oligodendrogliomas. We all know that even the Scandinavian group of Dr. Busch and Dr. Christensen called them oligodendrocytomas of the optic chiasm. Would you kindly refer to this?

Dr. Calvo: In the case of the spongioblastomas and the astrocytomas of the cerebellum and the oligodendrogliomas of the optic nerve I am afraid that I am not in agreement with the master, because I think that these tumours of which we demonstrated a few cases are derived from a special type of glial cells, that is located in the optic tracts, the brain stem and the cerebellum. These cells which are rare, are bipolar and normally form a sheet in relation with the pia mater. I think that these tumours are derived from this type of cells and they are not oligodendroglia but a sort of polar astrocyte. Now to call such a cell an astrocyte on morphological grounds is I think wrong because they do not look like a star, they look like a bipolar cell, so the tumour made up of these cells would be better called glioma of the glia polaris or polar or pilocytic glioma, but not astrocytoma. Then there is also a very important difference between the astrocytomas and those tumours which could be called polar gliomas or pilocytic type of gliomas. It is very difficult to find any relation of the expansions of the cytoplasm with the blood vessels. There are very long processes almost as wide as the nuclei and they appear to be completely indifferent to the blood vessels. This may be the reason why Hortega called them oligodendrocytes or oligodendrogliomas. But I could not find with either staining method in the chiasma, the optic tract or pons any very clear relation of these bipolar cells with the blood vessels or with the pial membrane. So I don't think that this tumour should necessarily be thought of as in relation with the blood vessels nor on the other hand should the lack of correlation with the blood vessels encourage us to classify these tumours as oligodendrogliomas. The type of nucleus is completely different from what we see in oligodendrogliomas or in the rest of the brain tissue.

Another point of importance is the distinction of these polar gliomas from the 2 cases presented by Dr. Rubinstein which are very similar to our case of the cerebellum. This is also a young girl, 14 years of age with only 4 months preoperativ symptoms and 6 months of survival. If we compare this with the many years of preoperative symptoms in Rubinstein's cases it is quite a different behaviour. Now in both cases, i. e. in my case here and both cases of Dr. Rubinstein we find this palisading and a greater relation of these cells to the blood vessels than was present in our case which could be considered an astroglioma. So the relation of these cells to the blood vessels could be a morphological feature for differentiating the two groups. In my case here I saw also many cells which were differentiated in the direction of astroblasts with silver impregnation. So one may be a sort of piloid or polar glioma and the other appear like a spongioblastoma with some differentiation in the direction of astroblastoma.

Dr. Zülch: I think this was a very important characteristic which Dr. Calvo has mentioned, the relation of the tumour cells to the blood vessels, as this is a point which we can follow with great difficulty in our usual routine aniline work but where the "impregnators" — if I may call them thus — have always an advantage. You remember our discussion last night on the foot plates of the astrocytes. May I propose here an extensive study be made on the foot plates in ependymomas, the so-called astroblastomas and in this type of spongioblastoma etc. And although most of us have neglected this in the last decade, we have perhaps to come back to silver work and do more extensive studies on our tumours according to methods which Dr. Calvo may recommend.

Dr. Calvo: That I do with pleasure I will send to every member of the Symposium a list of the methods as they are used in our laboratory.

Dr. Zülch: Dr. Rubinstein wants to say something.

Dr. Rubinstein: Yes, in agreement with Dr. Ringertz views, I think we are dealing with a separate entity. I also agree with Dr. Ringertz that the pilocytic appearance of the cells, the so-called bipolar appearance, is not to be ascribed in these cases to preexisting nerve tracts. My remarks were confined to the diffuse type of glioma infiltrating the pons in children which I think is an entirely different tumour.

The first point about Dr. Calvo's most interesting remarks is about the optic nerve tumours. This is a difficult subject and will lead us into a long discussion, but I would like to refer to a recent paper by Sarah Luse in the Journal of Neurosurgery * in which she did electron microscopy on an optic nerve glioma and on this evidence came to the conclusion that they were essentially astrocytomas. The second point concerns the pilocytic astrocytes. Here I don't follow the argument, because I see no objection to a mature astrocyte not being stellate. One does have reactive astrocytes in many neuropathological conditions which are pilocytic in form. That they have bipolar or unipolar processes does not prevent them from being mature. The same point I think is germane regarding the relation of the astrocyte to the blood vessel. Many astrocytes are not attached to blood vessels at all, many of them are attached to the lepto-meninges. You pointed out the relationship of these polar cells to the lepto-meniges in optic nerve glioma. I think this does not invalidate the concept that these are essentially astrocytes. I think that Dr. Calvo's case was originally a true polar spongioblastoma showing differentiation, much more than in our case, to both astroblastic and astrocytic forms. It would fall within the group described as showing transition towards astrocytoma. I would like to recall that these cases originally described by Dorothy Russell were seen by Hortega and he was the only one to offer a name for this tumour. He called it an astro-blastoma, because he did not accept the spongioblast as an entity and any primitive astrocyte was regarded by him as an astroblast.

Dr. Netsky: Listening to this conversation, I noticed an interesting phenom-enon and that is the tendency we have to slip sometimes from a histologic description to a clinical description. And I think again it is due to the misuse of the word malignancy which we use interchangeably for a clinical and his-tologic condition, but I think we would be much safer if we define our terms and were certain when we are talking that we are referring to the histologic malignancy as opposed to the clinical malignancy. I think we have to concede that a cerebral astrocytoma of exactly similar appearance may cause death in one patient, if it is situated in the frontal lobe, in a year and in another pa-tient in 5 years and this does not necessarily mean a different tumour from the histological standpoint, it may be different from the clinical standpoint, but we have to separate the two. I think also that Dr. Calvo makes a good point of defining an astrocyte as a star-shaped cell and a spongioblast as a polar cell, but I have to remind him that in the dynamic experiments, in the staining experiments one can show — I discussed that yesterday — that these may be interchangeable that one may go into the other and it depends on the conditions, the conditions of dilution, the conditions of compression, and as Dr. Ringertz already has emphasized that this is not the only factor, there may be other factors and many of them perhaps are unknown, may be chemical features, certainly the rate of growth in the individual cell, the existing dilution in the tissue as in the microcyst might already change it. So we have many factors that may change what appears to be an astrocyte to what appears to be a spongioblast and we are dealing with many unknown figures. I think we should keep that in mind.

Dr. Zülch: Thank you, Dr. Netsky.

---

* J. Neurosurg., Springfield, *18* (1961), 466—478.

Dr. Calvo: I would like to comment on the correlation of clinic and morphology and on the basis of the very important work of Dr. Netsky and Dr. Kersting. We may even question the justification for considering a tumour benign because a patient has been allowed to survive a few years. It will be better to say that if the patient lets the tumour live in his brain for a long time it will be a benign looking tumour, but if the patient allows the cells to develop rapidly it will look like a malignant tumour.

Dr. Zülch: That is a good remark. Dr. Müller wants to speak.

Dr. Müller: Dr. Kersting, have you seen in your explants Rosenthal fibres?

Dr. Kersting: No, not in culture.

Dr. Müller: Because we have noticed that according to Dietzel, the substances that are predominant in the Rosenthal fibres, are proteins and mucopolysaccharides and lipoids and we have shown that these substances do not stem from degeneration of the glia cell; we have seeen them absorbed from the neighbourhood and therefore the same substances can be seen in the gemistocytic astrocytes. Their contents may have the same histochemistry.

Dr. Zülch: Histochemically, I agree, Dr. Müller. But against you speaks the formation of Rosenthal fibres in the leptomeninges, because there are no myelin sheaths here and nothing else from which they could extract this material, you have found histochemically. Moreover, I think, one can histologically prove that true glial fibres are continuing into Rosenthal fibres (see Figure 81 d, Handbuch d. Neurochirurgie, Band III, Springer 1956). I can show this in Dr. Calvo's preparations and in Hortega's pictures.

Dr. Rubinstein: I can confirm the presence of Rosenthal fibers in the leptomeninges. It is conclusive evidence that they originate from the glial tumour cells themselves.

Dr. Calvo: I would like to make one more comment about Rosenthal fibres. I think that not every elongated fibre appearing as the only expansion of one cell should be called a Rosenthal fibre and many times, I think, we make this mistake. I saw many times in inflammatory reactions of the ependyma, proliferations of these glial epithelial cells with very long processes that are clearly coming from the glial epithelium. I think that these are true Rosenthal fibres.

Dr. Zülch: Well, I think the definition of Rosenthal fibres is clear in so far as no ordinary glial fibre of a cell in a bipolar spongioblastoma could be thus called. It is a particular product which is shown by various dyes best, one of the first being Heidenhain's haematoxylin. And they show up also in haematoxylin and eosin, where ordinarily you don't see glial fibres but you see the Rosenthal fibre stained reddish. Very often in impregnations you are able to see the continuation of one into the other, a true glial fibre into a Rosenthal fibre. So an ordinary glial fibre, even a thickened cell must not be called a Rosenthal fibre. Rosenthal fibre implies certain staining properties, which are well known.

Dr. Netsky: May I ask Dr. Zülch if he would make one modification concerning the origin of Rosenthal fibre by saying histologically proven, histologically inferred or histologically suggested?

Dr. Zülch: Well, I would say: I could show you the continuation of an impregnated glial fibre into a sausage-like product which corresponds to the definition of Rosenthal fibres. Is that clear now?

Dr. Rubinstein: I realized that the discussion on the polar spongioblastoma would inevitably lead to a discussion on Rosenthal fibres. Incidentally one is often asked what are Rosenthal fibres and one leads the person to the microscope, and he looks at the little bits of eosin and he says: "Oh, is that all?"

But I would like to refer to the question of their origin. It has been repeatedly suggested that they arise from the subependymal glia. Certainly as regards tumours there is some suggestive evidence. But I would refer to that remarkable series of cases which now seem to form an entity and are not tumours at all. These are the cases described by Alexander, by Crome, by Wohlwill and more recently in the subependymal glia, but around the blood vessels, throughout the brain and beneath the pia. Here you seem to have the same phenomenon but generalized throughout the neuroglial network and this raises the question as to whether these Rosenthal fibres are at all specific for subependymal glia. Would you like to comment?

Dr. Zülch: Yes, I have discussed that question very often with Dr. Hallervorden, and he thinks, that this is a failure in the migrating of the spongioblasts and he is of the opinion that ordinarily the formation of Rosenthal fibres is characteristic of the subependymal glia, but there are cases very often in Recklinghausen's or some other diseases where you have a failure in the migration of the various cells and then you have this type which we call subependymal glia all over the brain. This type of glia may be an entity, I don't know, we just name it after its primary location. When this form of glia is spread all over the brain, then you may have Rosenthal fibres through the whole hemisphere. That is my explanation of this.

Dr. Rubinstein: It may therefore be a phenomenon of what microscopists refer to as "surface glia", the glia which lines the ependymal surface, the meningeal surface and the Virchow-Robin space?

Dr. Zülch: Well, I don't know, I could not answer that question but certainly it has the characteristics of a specific form of glia.

Dr. Rubinstein: In optic nerve gliomas you may find a tremendous accumulation of Rosenthal fibres in close relation to the vascular stroma. It is reminiscent of the cases that Dr. Hallervorden has reviewed recently.

Dr. Zülch: I think there is a close relationship clinically between v. Recklinghausen's disease or at least the forme fruste of v. Recklinghausen's disease and the occurance of optic glioma. Very many of the patients who have these pigmentary naevi and the café au lait spots actually belong to formes frustes of v. Recklinghausen's disease. This has been clearly shown by Busch and Christensen in their work *.

Dr. Sayre: Someone working in our laboratories is reviewing spinal cord tumours and he reviewed some cases of syringomyelia associated with Rosenthal fibres in the syrinx. Are these also considered to be derived from subependymal cells?

Dr. Zülch: Yes. Actually the first description of Rosenthal was in a case of spinal ependymoma. The fibres were seen in the surroundings of the tumour. If you look at this picture, they were seen at the edge of the ependymoma and this developed as usually, in the dorsal part of the spinal cord. Probably it was the subependymal or pericanalicular glia which had reacted to the tumour growth by proliferation and thereby formation of Rosenthal fibres. You may see it for instance in a spinal angioblastoma at the boundary zone. Dr. Woolf and myself have recently seen them at the edge of a neurinoma near the IVth ventricle. Here the subventricular part will react to tumour growth or to compression or say to any sort of damage by proliferation and formation of Rosenthal fibres. They are not specific for any sort of blastomatous growth. It

---

* *Busch, E.,* and *E. Christensen,* Das Oligodendrocytom der Sehnervenkreuzung. Zbl. Neurochir. 2 (1937), 315—320.

is just one specific degenerative form of glia apparently, which may be either blastomatous — i. e. in a spongioblastoma — or periblastomatous.

Dr. Woolf: One question to Dr. Rubinstein about terminology. I think he suggested that we use a term "juvenile pilocytic astrocytoma" to distinguish it from certain other pilocytic astrocytomas and I thought you wanted also to include the benign hypertrophy of the pons. Or am I wrong?

Dr. Rubinstein: No, I said "so-called hypertrophy". This is the classical pontine glioma with which we are all familiar. I think the majority of these tumours are quite different from the group under discussion. These are diffuse and show no microcystic changes, but a remarkable tendency towards histological malignancy. It is possible of course that among the pontine tumours there are a small group of cases which are of the Bailey spongioblastoma type. But you will find described in a number of atlases pictures of the diffuse pontine glioma which does not belong into this category. And we tried to separate them from the Bailey type of spongioblastoma in our discussion. They are, I think, malignant astrocytomas of the pons with a tendency towards an anaplastic evolution.

Dr. Woolf: These are the ones that you say are pilocytic in the ventral parts and stellate in the tegmental.

Dr. Rubinstein: Yes, and I think in these cases the shape of the cells is virtually entirely due to the large number of fibre tracts, the central fibres diverging in one direction and the pyramidal tract in an other.

Dr. Woolf: They are also occur in the juvenile period?

Dr. Rubinstein: They are the common pontine gliomas of children often with a rather long clinical history which may suggest subacute encephalitis.

Dr. Woolf: Se we do have to be a little bit careful with your classification, that there are two types of juvenile fibrous astrocytoma.

Dr. Rubinstein: These are not juvenile types in the sense we have suggested. I used the term juvenile in an attempt to follow Dr. Zülch's suggestion that these are separate, and I would regard Bailey's polar spongioblastomas as the exact equivalent of the juvenile type. The pontine gliomas are a quite different clinico-pathological entity.

Dr. Woolf: And how do you refer to those?

Dr. Rubinstein: As malignant astrocytomas of the pons.

Dr. Netsky: May I have one suggestion for Dr. Rubinstein. Your original object was to obtain a classification and one most admirable virtue of a classification is some degree of consistency. When one introduces an age concept into a clinical pathological entity this is becoming inconsistant since we would always say an astrocytoma of a juvenile person is similar to an astrocytoma of an old person so that if we are using a nomenclature of this type we may discard the age as part of it. We may also find it occuring in 30 year old or 50 year old persons.

Dr. Zülch: Thank you, Dr. Netsky, this was a very good point.

IV. Polymorphous Oligodendroglioma

Chairman: The main subject of the day will he the definition of the oligo-dendroglioma particularly with regard to its possible polymorphous transformation and appearance. But I thought it would be appropriate to have as introduction the contribution of our member Dr. Rubinstein, who wishes to refer to the possibility of a mixed composition of tumours, particularly since in regard to the oligodendrogliomas the question may be raised whether they are true oligodendrogliomas or a mixture of oligodendrogliomas and astrocytomas. Therefore it might be quite a good introduction to have Dr. Rubinstein's speech first.

Morphological Problems of Brain Tumors with Mixed Cell Population

By

L. J. Rubinstein

With 18 Figures

The present classifications of tumors of the glioma group are based, like those of neoplasms elsewhere in the body, on the recognition of the morphological characteristics of the prevalent cell component. The existence has, however, long been recognized, in many cases, of a diversity in cell population which cannot reasonably be explained by a process of anaplastic degradation of the more differentiated glial elements. This discussion will be concerned with three different, and unrelated, aspects of this problem. The first is presented by tumors composed of more than one gliogenous element, often of adult form, and in which it cannot be argued that any one cell type is derived from another *(mixed gliomas)*. The second bears on the rare group of ganglion-cell tumors of the central nervous system, in which both neuronal and glial elements can be demonstrated to participate in the neoplastic process *(gangliogliomas)*. The third aspect concerns those composite tumors in which, by analogy with the "carcinosarcomas" found elsewhere in the body, a mixture of both sarcomatous and gliomatous elements are found in contiguity *(mixed gliomas and sarcomas)*.

1. In the first group to be discussed, a lack of homogeneity in cellular composition is widely acknowledged. This diversity is, for example, abundantly reflected in the experimental work of *Zimmerman* and his colleagues [21] on the induction of cerebral gliomas in mice, as Dr. *Netsky* has recalled in the earlier discussions of this Symposium. In human material, this mixture may either be of an intimate kind or reveal a sharp transition of one glial type to another, which may sometimes be detected even with the naked eye. Perhaps the most frequent instance of this is exemplified by the foci

of gemistocytic appearance present in diffuse fibrillary cerebral astrocytomas. Another example is provided by the common participation of astrocytes or their precursors in the oligodendrogliomas, and of neoplastic oligodendroglia in cerebral astrocytomas, the extent of which is usually best revealed by the use of metallic techniques; this aspect has been developed at length in the studies of *Rio-Hortega* [12], *Ravens* and coll.[10], and many others. Distinct foci of oligodendroglioma have also been recognized in ependymomas, confirmed by silver impregnations in some cases [8]. They may also be found in a number of pilocytic astrocytomas of the cerebellum and in optic nerve gliomas. It is true that both *Zülch* [22] and *Ringertz* [11] have interpreted these foci as indicative of degeneration in the cells of tumors which they have labelled "polar spongioblastomas", but their ballooned appearance, recalling the "acute swelling" of normal oligodendroglia in post-mortem material, renders such foci indistinguishable, in our view, from those observed in otherwise typical oligodendrogliomas. These issues, based on conflicting morphological interpretations, are particularly reflected in the case of the optic nerve gliomas, where the variable patterns formed by the intimate mixture of piloid and stellate astrocytes with microcystic areas containing nests of vacuolated oligodendroglial cells have given rise, in the literature, to a variety of labels ranging from oligodendroglioma [1, 13] to astrocytoma [4] and spongioblastoma [22].

An illustration of this aspect, remarkable by its rarity, is provided in Fig. 1, from a fourth ventricle tumor of mixed cytology which had invaded the cerebellum and the leptomeninges in a child. In this field, two juxtaposed areas of different histological appearances are demonstrated: on the left, the distinctive architecture of the rare polar spongioblastoma as defined by *Russell* and *Cairns* [15], characterized by a conspicuous palisading of fine spongioblastic nuclei; on the right, the classical microcystic appearance of an oligodendroglioma. In this case (which I owe to the courtesy of Dr. *R. M. Norman,* Bristol), a silver carbonate impregnation confirmed the distinction between the spongioblastic and the oligodendroglial elements, fine glial fibrils and also immature astrocytes being easily identifiable amongst the former only. It may be added that these morphological appearances cannot be attributed to the presence of preexisting structures determining the alignment of the tumor cells, since the oligodendroglial component was entirely intraneural and the polar spongioblastoma largely intraventricular.

This, and other, examples illustrate a cytological variability which is not to be confused with the polymorphism associated with anaplasia, or dedifferentiation. In extreme instances such varieties may defy classification; in others a composite label, such as oligo-astrocytoma, may be devised for them as suggested by some authors; in many the convenience of naming the tumor by its prevalent cell type is maintained despite the recognition of its cellular diversity; or, in certain cases, a distinctive label may be appropriate in denoting a specific histological entity: the latter is exemplified in the "subependymoma" of *Scheinker* [18] a well-known variant of the ependymoma, in which an intimate mixture of ependymal cells with a densely fibrillary and sparsely cellular astrocytomatous

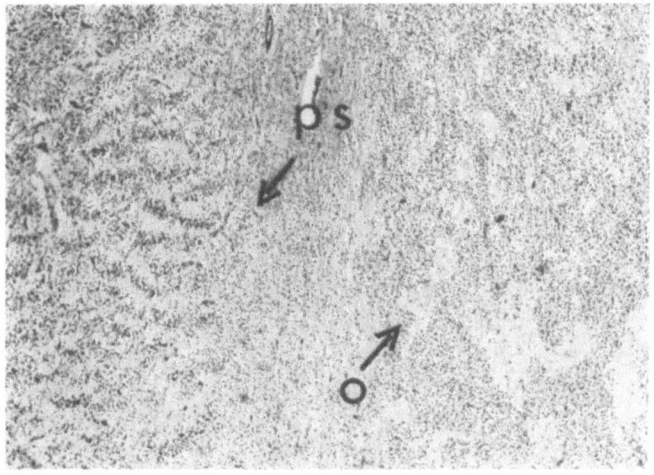

Fig. 1. Mixed glioma. On the left, polar spongioblastoma (ps) with typical arrangement in palisades. On the right, oligodendroglioma (o) with microcystic change. H. and E. 42 ×.

element derived from the subependymal neuroglia constitutes the characteristic feature.

2. The second group of neoplasms to be considered, the ganglion-cell tumors of the central nervous system, present a mixture of cell population which is of particular interest. These tumors are both rare and controversial. There is much dispute over their definition, nomenclature and biological behavior. Because of the frequent participation of neuroglial elements in the neoplastic process, we have subscribed to the concept introduced by *Courville* [2], according to which these tumors have been labelled gangliogliomas. The glial component is for the most part astrocytic, being constituted in some cases by uni- and bipolar pilocytic cells and in others by plump gemistocytic astrocytes. However, the extent to which the glia displays a neoplastic evolution may vary from case to case. In some, it is so

scanty that the tumor may be called a pure ganglioneuroma, or gangliocytoma. In others, neoplastic proliferation of the neuroglia may overshadow the neuronal element, so that the first microscopic impression is that of an astrocytoma. Intermediate grades between these two extremes are, however, most frequently encountered, i. e. gangliogliomas in which the neuronal and glial components are mingled in approximately equal proportions. In such cases, the cytological differentiation of one cell type usually parallels that of the other. But exceptions to this rule occasionally occur, and this

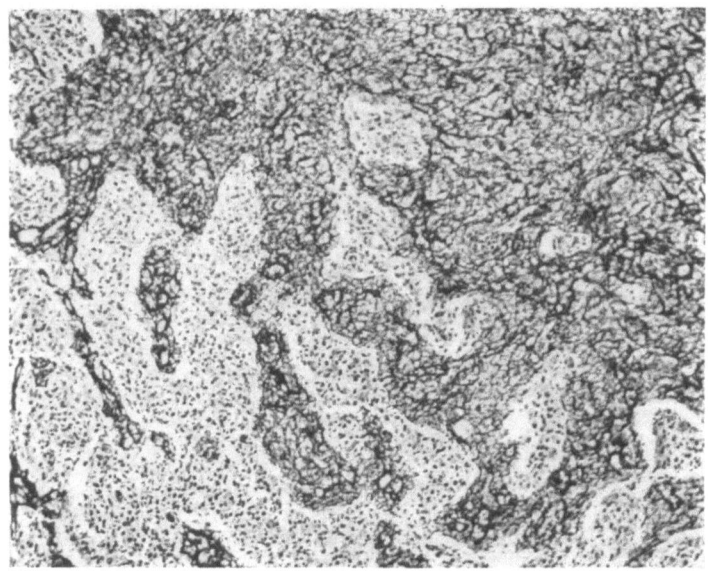

Fig. 2. Mixed sarcoma and glioma. Case 1. Edge of tumor, showing darkly staining reticulin-rich sarcoma forming irregular tongues which encompass clear, reticulin-free gliomatous islands
Gomori's reticulin stain 59 ×.

variability is of importance when their biological potentiality is assessed.

These neoplasms are usually, and justifiably, regarded as relatively benign and slowly-growing. The possible advent of a malignant change in these tumors introduces the obvious cytological and biological problem concerning the respective participation of the neuronal and neuroglial elements in this process. In the literature, malignant features have at times been reported (*Kernohan* and coll., case 3; *Tönnis* and *Zülch*, case 4)[9, 20], and it has been suggested that such a transformation is essentially the prerogative of the ganglion cells[3]. So definite an interpretation must, however, be open to question. Admittedly, if it is accepted that cells of ganglionic origin are capable of neoplastic proliferation at all, there can be no theoretical objection to the view that, on occasion, this proliferation might undergo an anaplastic evolution. But here we are confronted by the diagnostic difficulty that cells of this type would by the same token be deprived of most of their distinguishing neuronal hallmarks. Thus a confusion is particularly liable to arise in a rare form of highly malignant glioblastoma in which giant pyramidal cells of ganglionic appearance may be a conspicuous feature. In this type of cell, Nissl substance and neurofibrils cannot be demon-

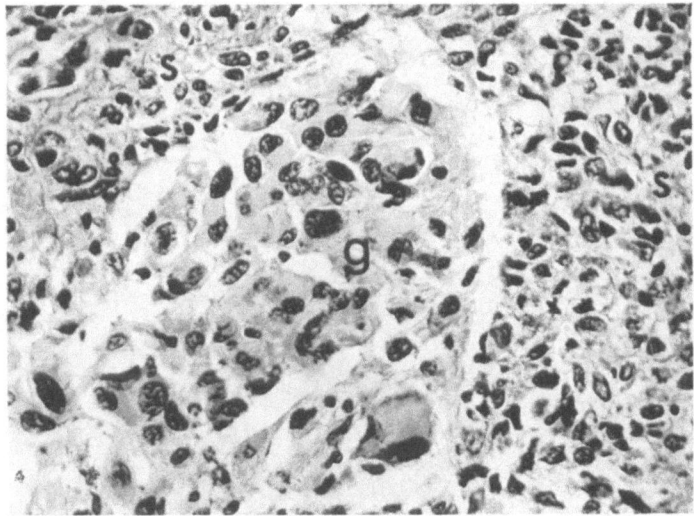

Fig. 3. Case 1. High-power view of gliomatous island (g) surrounded on either side by sarcoma cells (s). Van Gieson 330 ×.

strated, and all transitional forms to other anaplastic elements of neuroglial origin can usually be traced.

From our knowledge, therefore, of the respective potential activities of both ganglionic and glial cells, and by analogy with the known behavior of many cerebral astrocytomas, it might be supposed *a priori* that anaplastic changes in the glia would be more probable. In two distances of ganglioglioma from our own material we have noted anaplastic cellular features which appeared referable entirely to the glial element, and we have therefore suggested that when they undergo a malignant change it is in the latter, and not in the neuronal element, that this is usually witnessed (*Russell* and *Rubinstein,* p. 168) [16]. A more recently investigated example supports this view with particular clarity.

This case is that of a woman who, following a two years' history of increased intracranial pressure, underwent at the age of 26 the partial removal of an intraventricular tumor arising from the lateral wall of the left frontal horn. Microscopically this revealed a poorly cellular ganglioglioma of benign appearance. Fourteen years later, progressive clinical symptoms indicative of a gradual recurrence of the tumor became manifest, ultimately leading to the patient's death 23 years after the original operation. Autopsy confirmed the re-currence of a tumor obliterating the body and anterior horn of the left lateral ventricle, with an extensive caudal extension, along the

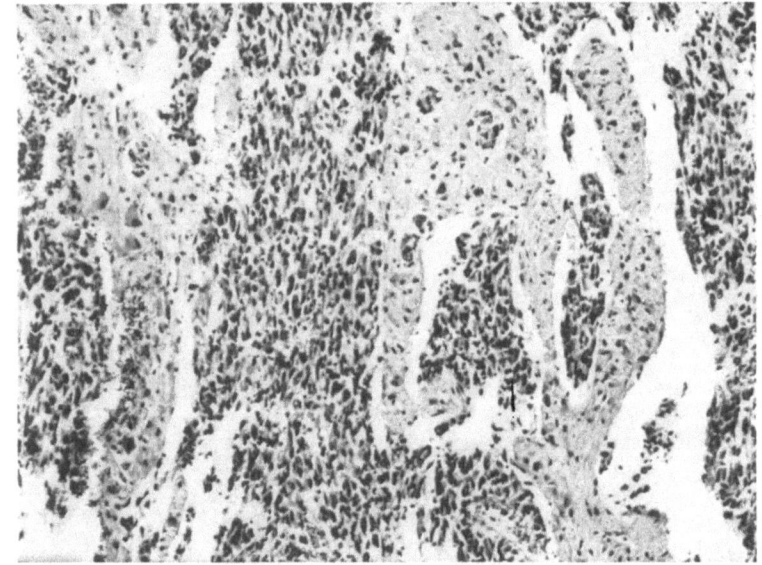

Fig. 4. Case 1. Another part of the tumor. Tongues of darkly staining sarcoma cells irregularly infiltrating paler glial tissue showing atypical reactive gliosis. H. and E. 90 ×.

corpus callosum and other median structures, which fanned out posteriorly into the medial halves of both occipital lobes. Here the appearances recalled a classical glioblastoma multiforme. The micro-scopic appearances of the intraventricular tumor located antero-laterally were essentially similar to those of the biopsy removed 23 years previously, namely those of a ganglion-cell tumor without histological evidence of anaplasia; whereas those of its contiguous, more medially located portion displayed, on proceeding more cau-dally, the progressively malignant features of an infiltrating astro-cytoma dedifferentiating into a glioblastoma.

The interest of this case, more fully reported elsewhere [17], lies in the long survival of the patient (23 years) from the time of her first operation. The clinical symptomatology, manifested over a span of 25 years, and the pathological findings disclosed on two widely separated occasions, permit us to reconstruct the lines of the tumor's evolution: they would indicate that extremely slow growth, with possibly long intervals of arrest and accompanied by continuous differentiation of the neuronal element, constituted the main feature of the original centrally located ganglioglioma. This benign evolution was overtaken, in the later stages, by a widespread acceleration of the neoplastic process, now accompanied by anaplasia, in which participation of only the glial element was

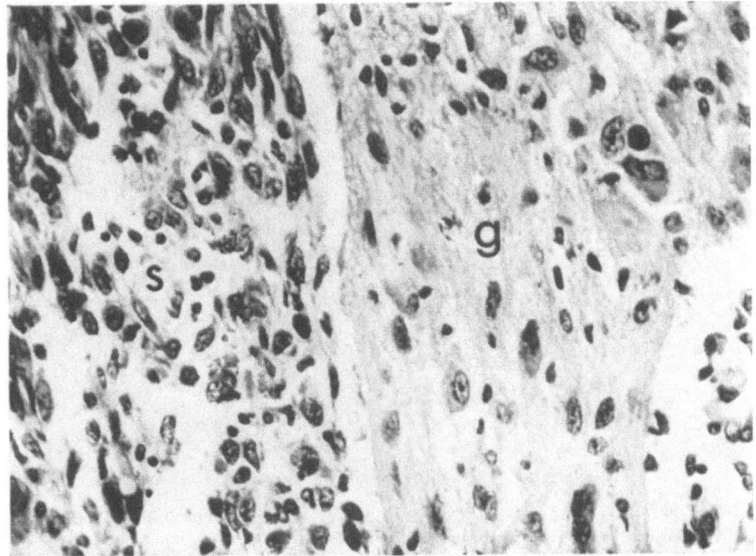

Fig. 5. Case 1. High-power view of Fig. 4. Reactive glia with atypical cytological features (g), contiguous to sheet of anaplastic sarcoma cells (s). H. and E. 330 ×.

demonstrated. The picture of a massive glioblastoma multiforme was thus ultimately produced.

3. In the last few years, interest has been revived in the existence of mixed or composite sarcomatous and gliomatous brain tumors, a concept originally implied in the term "gliosarcoma" introduced by *Stroebe* [19] in 1895, but for which no place has, up until now, been provided in modern classifications. Nonetheless, some thirty tumors of this kind have now been reported in the literature, and we have had the opportunity to examine, at the London Hospital, fifteen such examples, many of which were referred to us from elsewhere. The development of mixed tumors in which these two types of tissue lie in juxtaposition is assumed to originate in two different

forms. In the first, and by far the smaller, group, accounting for four cases in our material, the tumor appears to be primarily a meningeal sarcoma or a malignant meningioma, whose invasion of the brain is accompanied by a vigorous proliferative and hyperplastic reaction of the surrounding neuroglia, in which cytologically neoplastic features are demonstrated. The appearances then are those of a central sarcoma with a peripheral zone of glioma. Such an event is illustrated in Fig. 2 to 5, from a well-circumscribed cystic parietal tumor in a woman of 60 (courtesy of Dr. *D. R. Oppenheimer,* Oxford). Fig. 2, taken from the periphery of the growth,

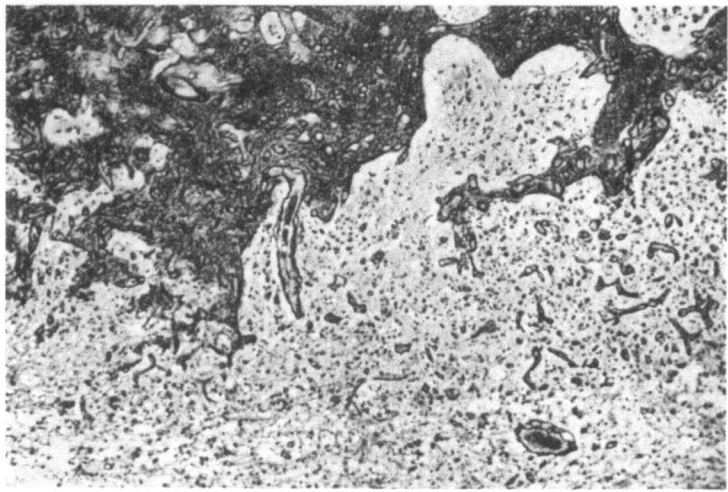

Fig. 6. Mixed sarcoma and glioma. Case 2. Edge of tumor: darkly staining reticulin-rich sarcoma irregularly invading a grey zone of glioma. The paler greyish band along the lower edge of the photograph shows non-neoplastic reactive gliosis only. Foot's reticulin method 69 ×

illustrates in a low-power field stained for reticulin the irregular invasion of the brain by fibroblastic tumor with the segregation of pale glial islands within its borders. Fig. 3 demonstrates, at a higher power, the contrasting cytology of a gliomatous island encompassed by sarcoma cells. Elsewhere, the sarcomatous tumor was sharply demarcated from a peripheral zone of densely cellular gliomatous tissue exhibiting in places an early pseudo-palisading of the nuclei around small foci of necrosis, characteristic of glioblastoma. A further histological feature of this case was the demonstration, from field to field, of a variable intensity in the malignant change of the glial element, with transitional stages ranging from atypical hyperplasia to frank neoplasia. Figs. 4 and 5 illustrate one of these transitional zones, in which the advancing tongues of sarcoma cells enclose paler glial islands exhibiting a considerably lesser degree of malignancy, but in which individual cell elements already show evidence of atypical changes.

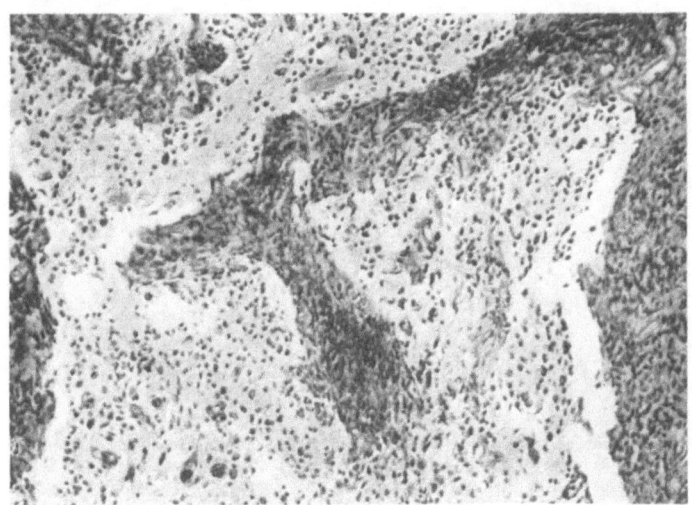

Fig. 7. Case 2 Cellular features, at low power, of the edge of the sarcoma. Darkly-staining tongues of sarcoma sprouting into paler zones of cellular glioma. Van Gieson 100 ×.

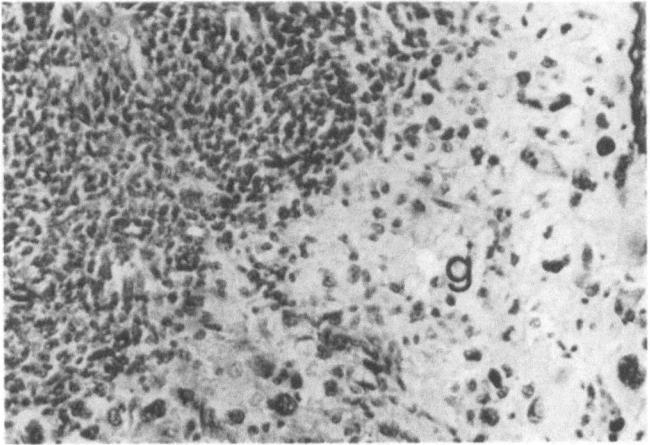

Fig. 8. Case 2. Contrasting cytology of compact sarcoma cells (s) in upper left half of field, contiguous to looser anaplastic glial cells (g) in lower right half. Van Gieson 180 ×.

The questions raised by this neoplastic alteration of the surrounding glia secondary to an invasive mesodermal tumor are of obvious interest in the context of the pathogenesis of tumor in-

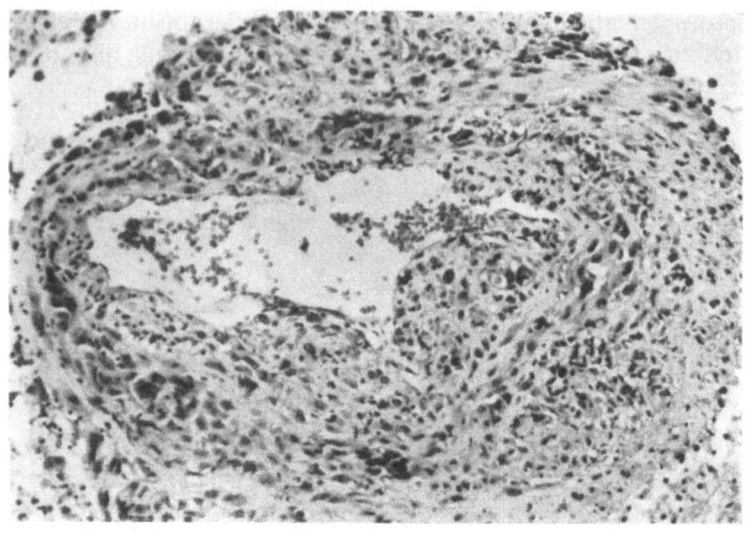

Fig. 9. Mixed glioma and sarcoma. Case 3. Blood vessel showing intravascular and perivascular
proliferation with malignant cytological features. H. and E. 135 ×.

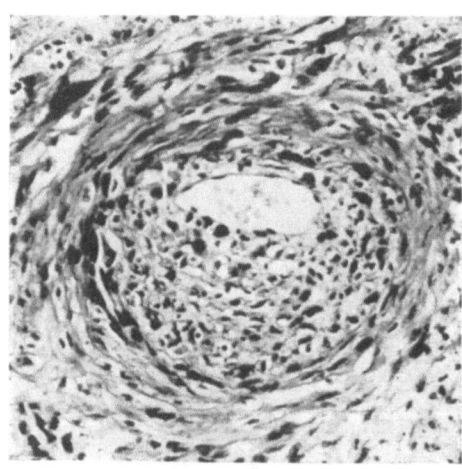

Fig. 10. Case 3. Malignant cytological features in
endothelial proliferation of another blood vessel,
with fusiform periadventitial cells radiating off
the vessel wall. Van Gieson 155 ×.

duction in general. Such a malignant glial reaction seems to have its counterpart in other neoplasms, where the term "collateral hyperplasia" has been coined to describe the proliferation of invaded tissues in the vicinity of epithelial tumors. According to *Ewing*[5] this may present as hypertrophy, hyperplasia and atypicality of the lining cells, which may approach the appearances of carcinoma and may be scarcely distinguishable from it, as seen, for example, in the atypical proliferation of acini in adrenals invaded by renal carcinoma. It is of interest that the malignant glial reaction to an invasive mesodermal brain tumor of the character described above may remain localized to the macroscopic margin of the growth. This was noted in a previously recorded case (*Rubinstein,* case 2)[14], in which a spindle-cell sarcoma of the leptomeninges was surgically excised from a 21 year-old woman. The microscopic appearances demonstrating the neoplastic glial reaction contiguous to the invasive sarcoma are illustrated in Figs. 6 to 8. Extirpation of the tumor has been followed by an apparently successful cure, the patient being now perfectly well ten years after surgery.

In the second, and larger, group of composite sarcomatous and gliomatous neoplasms, the sarcomatous changes have apparently arisen from the pronounced vascular proliferation so characteristi-

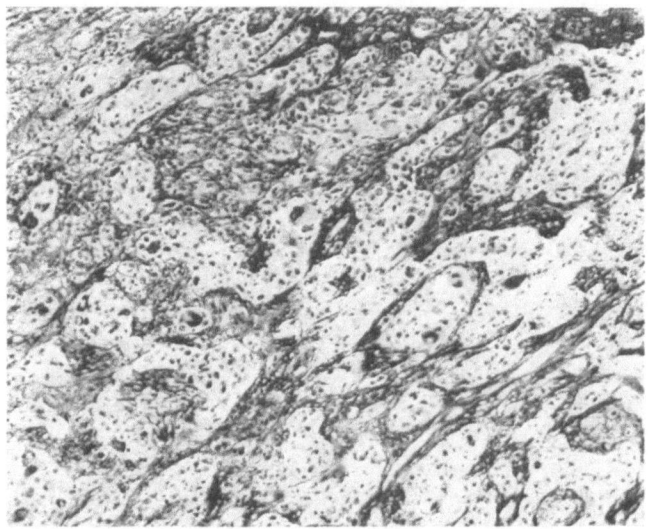

Fig. 11. Case 3. Characteristic marmorate pattern produced by pale gliomatous islands, containing giant cells, enclosed by bands of darkly staining fibroblastic tissue. Van Gieson 69 ✕.

cally found in glioblastomas. This phenomenon has been well studied by *Feigin* and his colleagues [6, 7]. We have now seen eleven cases in which this interpretation seems valid. The full development of this process is certainly rare, and has been estimated by *Feigin* to occur in about 2% of gliomas. But when a large series of glioblastomas is systematically examined, transitional features between hyperplastic and frankly neoplastic vascular proliferations are not infrequently encountered, producing in some cases a complete obliteration of the lumen by plump, hyperchromatic spindle cells. The acquisition, by the endothelial and fibroblastic advential cells, of obviously malignant features such as atypical mitoses, conspicuous nuclear polymorphism and multinucleated giant cells, marks a further stage in this neoplastic evolution. Surrounding the walls of these atypical blood vessels, and apparently arising from them, thick collars of large fusiform cells are formed which fan out further afield to merge into zones of spindle-cell sarcoma and fibro-sarcoma. The sarcomatous sheets then appear to "invade" the glio-matous tissue, producing in places a characteristic marmorate pattern. The wealth of reticulin fibrils, strictly limited to the sar-comatous areas, provides a sharp contrast to the adjacent glioma;

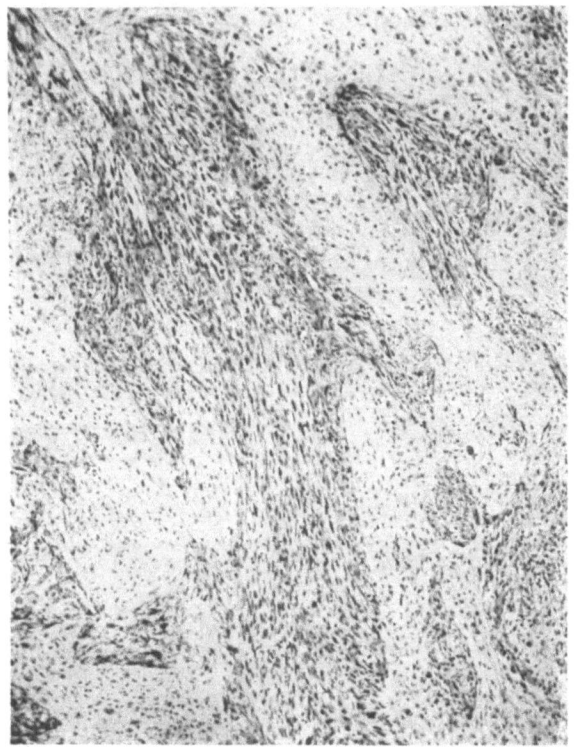

Fig. 12. Case 3. Darkly staining fibrosarcomatous sheets separated by pale gliomatous zones.
Van Gieson 58 ×.

the two types of tissue are furthermore readily recognized by the Van Gieson method, where the looser texture of the pale glial zones, exhibiting plump astrocytic elements, is easily contrasted with the more darkly staining and compact architecture of the fibroblastic sarcoma; or by the PTAH stain which, by the specific staining of neuroglial fibrils, confirms the identity of the gliomatous com-ponent. These features are illustrated in Figs. 9 to 13, from a well-circumsribed, very firm lobulated tumor with central necrosis, un-

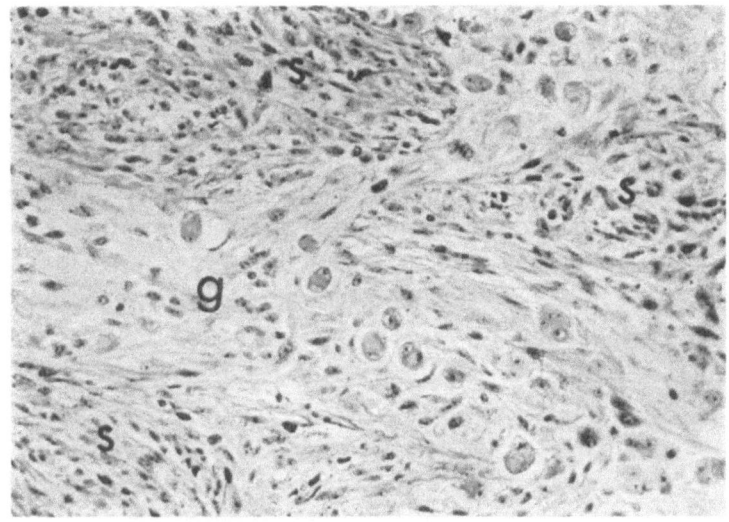

Fig. 13. Case 3. Cytological detail of central gliomatous zone (g) bordered by more compact fibrosarcomatous areas (s). Mallory's P. T. A. H. 185 ×.

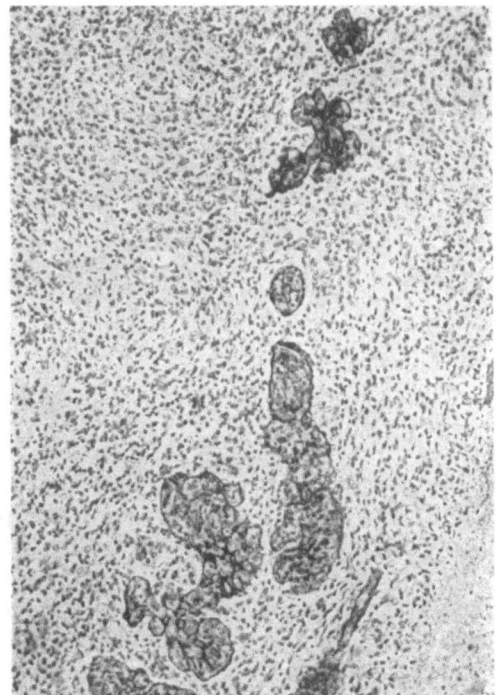

Fig. 14. Case 4. Mixed glioma and sarcoma. Original biopsy. Areas of glioblastoma with typical "glomerular" formations of vascular endothelial proliferation. Foot's reticulin method 73 ×.

attached to the dura, and removed from the right temporal lobe of
a man of 48. This example, which outwardly mimicked a meningioma, is more fully reported elsewhere (*Rubinstein,* case 4)[14].

Biologically these tumors behave essentially like highly malignant glioblastomas, and display a most rapid growth rate. The
sarcomatous change, though regarded as a secondary phenomenon
often gives the impression of occuring *pari passu* with the growth

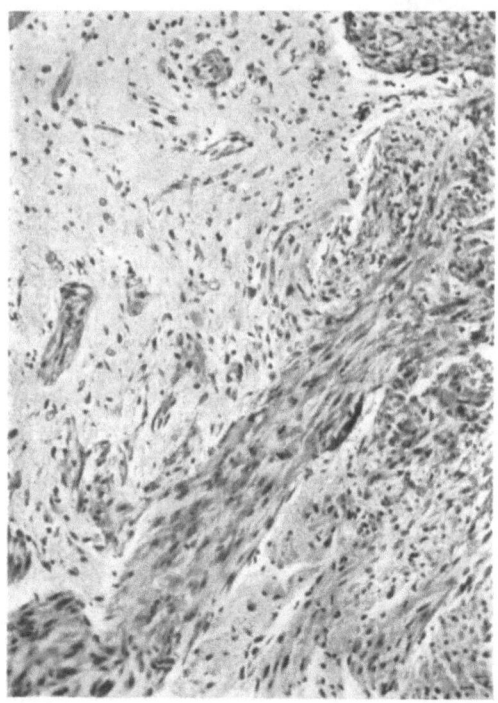

Fig. 15. Case 4. Original biopsy. Zone of sarcoma sprouting into the adjacent cortex. The latter
shows reactive gliosis only. Van Gieson 100 ×.

and spread of the glioma. Often, the change is focal and microscopic only; or only a relatively early stage of this process may be
seen in the blood vessel walls, though the histological appearances
are already unequivocal. Rarely such a focus may be detected
macroscopically as a circumscribed nodule of pale, woody hard
consistency in an otherwise typical glioblastoma. It should be
stressed that the cytology and histological architecture of such a
fibrosarcomatous focus differ altogether from the elements of
organizing granulation tissue which are commonly found as a re-

action to an old necrosis in a glioblastoma. Furthermore, it may happen that the sarcoma reaches such massive proportions that the glioma is almost entirely overshadowed. Such an example is demonstrated in Figs. 14 to 18, from a left posterior temporal tumor attached to the tentorium, partly removed from a man of 49 with a three year history of gradual mental deterioration. Biopsy fragments displayed a mixture of sarcomatous and gliomatous elements, as illustrated in Figs. 14 and 15. Six months after the operation, the patient died with a massive left temporal recurrence, the ventral half of which, as demonstrated in Fig. 16, presented at necropsy as a woody hard, lobulated growth with a circumscribed outline.

Microscopically, the appearances were now largely those of a perivascular fibrosarcoma (Figs. 17 and 18). Though many areas of this tumor were submitted to histological examination, only one small portion was found to disclose its essentially gliomatous origin; this would perhaps have been even more difficult to establish were it not for the clear evidence obtained from the biopsy performed six months before death.

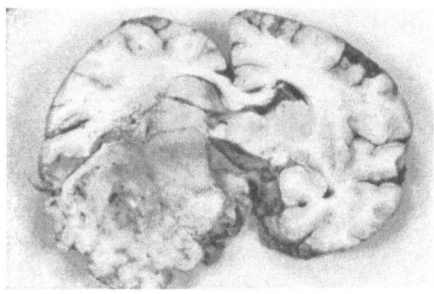

Fig. 16. Case 4. Necropsy specimen. Massive recurrence of a left temporal tumor, the ventral portion of which was woody hard and markedly lobulated.

It may thus become apparent that these mixed tumors have from the morphological standpoint a possible, and in some cases a definite, relationship with the "circumscribed sarcomas arising from the blood vessels" or "monstrocellular sarcomas" described by *Zülch* [22]. Though marked resemblances are certainly met between the examples described above and those he has illustrated, and though our own cases too exhibit in places large numbers of giant and even monster cells, a definite equation of both entities is not yet wholly warranted, since some of the cases described and illustrated by *Zülch* display histological features which are quite at variance with the examples now under discussion.

It is of course realized that the problem of the classification of brain tumors is hardly facilitated by an undue emphasis on those examples which display an obvious mixture of cell population. The object of these brief considerations has, however, been to draw attention to the existence of recognizable morphological entities, however difficult they may be to fit into existing schemes or nomen-

clatures. The conclusions hereby suggested may be summarized as
follows:

1. In the glioma group, the existence of cases with a mixed cell
population is not necessarily an impediment to any workable classification, since, as originally stressed by *Bailey,* the obligation is accepted of labelling a glioma by its prevalent cell type. However, the

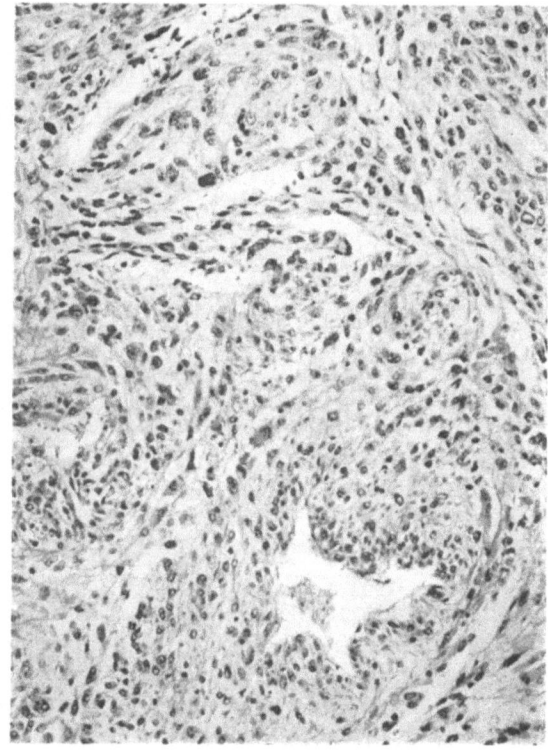

Fig. 17. Case 4. Microscopic appearances of the tumor necropsy, showing the cytological features
of a perivascular fibrosarcoma. Van Gieson 120 ×.

presence, widely acknowledged, of mixed cell types in many, if not
most, tumors merits emphasis as constituting an important morphological factor in determining in part their biological behavior. The
identification of cell mixtures of *adult* forms must clearly be distinguished from the concept of cellular anaplasia or dedifferentiation.
Moreover, the supervention of anaplasia in a glioma with an originally mixed cell population results in a further blurring of the
neat boundaries of our taxonomic conventions. That neuroonco-
logists should thus be confronted by the pleomorphism and bio-

logical variabilities of hitherto accepted tumor entities is therefore not surprising: hence the morphological and semantic confusion reflected in our highly artificial, and sometimes conflicting, schemes of classification.

2. In ganglion-cell tumors the presence of mixed ganglionic and glial cell forms is of more than merely academic interest, since

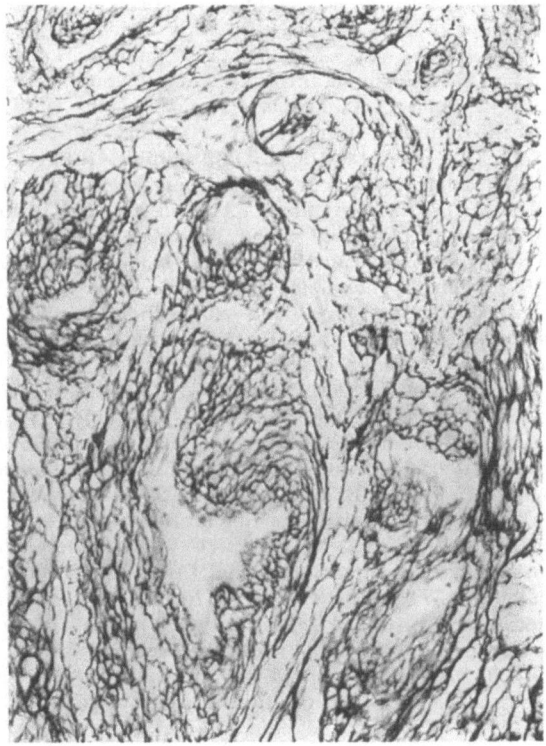

Fig. 18. Case 4. Similar field to Fig. 17, stained for reticulin (perivascular fibrosarcoma). Gomori's reticulin 110 ×.

it is suggested that in such cases the glial element only is the one susceptible of a malignant evolution.

3. The presence of mixed gliomas and sarcomas, hitherto unacknowledged in modern schemes of classification, appears accountable by

    a) either a malignant change in the neuroglia adjacent to an invasive sarcoma,

    b) or a sarcomatous change arising from the vascular proliferations so commonly encountered in glioblastomas. The impression gained is that the second interpretation is by far the more likely one in most examples of this rare conjunction. The problem appears to be of considerable interest in the context of the pathogenesis of tumor induction in general.

References

1. *Christensen, E.*, and *S. R. Andersen*, Primary Tumors of the Optic Nerve and Chiasm. Acta psychiatr. neurol., K'hvn, 27 (1952), 5. — 2. *Courville, C. B.*. Ganglioglioma, Tumor of the Central Nervous System. Arch. Neurol. Psychiatr., Chicago, 24 (1930), 439. — 3. *Courville, C. B.*, and *K. H. Abbott*, Malignant Changes in Cerebral Ganglioglioma. Proc. Second. Int. Congr. Neuropath., London, 1 (1955), 105. — 4. *Davis, F. A.*, Primary Tumors of the Optic Nerve (a phenomenon of Recklinghausen's Disease). Arch. Ophthal., N. Y., 23 (1940), 735. — 5. *Ewing, J.*, Neoplastic diseases. 4th ed. Philadelphia, 1940. — 6. *Feigin, I. H.*, and *S. W. Gross*, Sarcoma Arising in Glioblastoma of Brain. Amer. J. Path. 31 (1955), 663. — 7. *Feigin, I.*, *L. B. Allen*, *L. Lipkin* and *S. W. Gross*, The Endothelial Hyperplasia of the Cerebral Blood Vessels with Brain Tumors and its Sarcomatous Transformation. Cancer, 11 (1958), 264. — 8. *Kernohan, J. W.*, and *E. M. Fletcher-Kernohan*. Ependymomas. A Study of 109 Cases. Res. Publ. Ass. Nerv. Ment. Dis., N. Y., 16 (1935), 182. — 9. *Kernohan, J. W.*, *J. R. Learmonth* and *J. B. Doyle*, Neuroblastomas and Gangliocytomas of the Central Nervous System. Brain, London, 55 (1932), 287. — 10. *Ravens, J. R.*, *L. L. Adamkiewicz* and *R. Groff*, Cytology and Cellular Pathology of the Oligodendrogliomas of the Brain. J. Neuropath., Baltimore, 14 (1955), 142. — 11. *Ringertz, N.*, and *H. Nordenstam*, Cerebellar astrocytoma. J. Neuropath., Baltimore, 10 (1951), 343. — 12. *Rio-Hortega, P. del.*, Contribucion al conocimiento citologico de los oligodendrogliomas. Arch. histol., B. Aires, 2 (1944), 266. — 13. *Rio-Hortega, P. del.*, Contribucion al conocimiento citologico de los tumores del nervio y quiasma optiquos. Arch. histol., B. Aires, 2 (1944), 307. — 14. *Rubinstein, L. J.*, The Development of Contiguous Sarcomatous and Gliomatous Tissue in Intracranial Tumours. J. Path. Bact. 71 (1956), 441. — 15. *Russell, D. S.*, and *H. Cairns*, Polar Spongioblastomas. Arch. histol., B. Aires, 3 (1947), 423. — 16. *Russell, D. S.*, and *L. J. Rubinstein*, Pathology of Tumours of the Nervous System. Edw. Arnold London, 1959. — 17. *Russell, D. S.*, and *L. J. Rubinstein*, Ganglioglioma: A Case with Long History and Malignant Evolution. J. Neuropath., Baltimore, 21 (1962), 185. — 18. *Scheinker, I. M.*, Subependymoma: A Newly Recognized Tumor of Subependymal Derivation. J. Neurosurg., Springfield, 2 (1945), 232. — 19. *Stroebe, H.*, Über Entstehung und Bau der Hirngliome. Beitr. path. Anat., Jena, 18 (1895). 405. — 20. *Tönnis, W.*, and *K. J. Zülch*, Intrakranielle Ganglienzellgeschwülste. Zbl. Neurochir. 4 (1939), 273. — 21. *Zimmerman, H. M.*, The Nature of Gliomas as Revealed by Animal Experimentation. Amer. J. Path. 31 (1955), 1. — 22. *Zülch, K. J.*, Biologie und Pathologie der Hirngeschwülste, Handbuch der Neurochirurgie, edited by *H. Olivecrona* and *W. Tönnis*, Springer, Berlin, vol. 3.

Discussion

Dr. Zülch: Dr. Rubinstein, we thank you very much for this most interesting and inspiring paper and in spite of your introductory remarks that it is not a good introduction to our discussion of polymorphous oligodendrogliomas, I think it was. But it goes far beyond this, you have raised a good many very important and I think basic questions of tumour terminology and classification and you have also touched on a good many problems of tumour pathogenesis. We won't be able to discuss most of your important problems and questions extensively during this meeting. But I expect they will give rise to an object for our next meeting maybe of the pathogenesis of tumours, and then, I think, the question of mixed tumours must play a very great part in our discussion. But there will be a lot of minor questions which we can discuss and quite a few of the major questions which we can at least try to tackle and I hope you will all want to say something about Dr. Rubinstein's paper, which is open now to discussion. I call Dr. Netsky.

Dr. Netsky: I am of course very pleased to hear this discussion because there is no inherent difficulty for me in understanding the problem of mixed tumours and so I am emphasizing the experimental work, most often experimental tumours are indeed mixed. I cannot help observing that there is a saying that seeing is believing but there is also the reverse and that is, we see what we believe. We believe tumours arise from a single cell and tumours are therefore uniform and we then make these diagnoses. This is common among the members of the committe or group here, I try to emphasize and I should like to reemphasize that this is rather arbitrary and these mixtures are probably more prevalent than we believe and they may even be universal, but we sometimes refuse to recognize it. I should like to submit that the pathogenesis of the glial tumours is by origin from multiple cells rather then from single cells. And I think, this represents a step along.

Dr. Sayre: I am likewise pleased to hear the discussion bring out this problem of mixed cellular types of gliomas. The experience that I have had suggested that there are a great number of oligodendrogliomas that are mixed with ependymal cells or astrocytic cells. Sometimes we call a tumour an ependymoma with astrocytes or an astrocytoma with ependymal cells and term it a mixed ependymoma-astrocytoma. Based on the same training and knowledge as Dr. Netsky in general pathological statements it is quite easy for me to envisage tumours made of two types of cells without necessarily saying that one is the reaction to another. And certainly in many of the ependymomas of the brain it is quite difficult to be sure as to whether one should make a diagnosis of ependymoma or astrocytoma because of the presence of the two types of cells. And this will come up again in the discussion of the oligodendrogliomas and the mixed nature of these particular types of tumours.

Dr. Zülch: Thank you, Dr. Sayre.

Dr. Ringertz: Among the many interesting questions Dr. Rubinstein took up in his paper there is only one in which I have some personal experience — the occurrence of "oligodendrogliomatous" looking areas in other tumours, especially ependymomas, spongioblastomas of the cerebellum and also in some cases of medulloblastoma. And I decided, and I have written this in my paper, that in my opinion these are degenerative cell changes. I based this opinion first on the fact that it is well known that this honeycomb picture of oligodendroglioma in fact is not a vital phenomenon, it is known that the better fixed the tissue is the less pronounced is the honeycomb pattern of an oligodendroglioma and so if you look upon the border zone of an oligodendroglioma, you often don't find this honeycomb pattern, you find it in the centre of the tumour, where perhaps the fixative has not gone in so very quickly. Now I think the proof of the presence of oligodendrocytes is easily obtained by impregnation. Let me say that I tried that, but unfortunately the material where I observed such areas was paraffin-embedded material with the inherent difficulty of showing with a special stain that the cells are oligodendrocytes. But I am quite ready to accept proof by other scientists by impregnation that oligodendrocytes are really present in such patches of oligodendroglioma-like tissues in other tumours, I will agree and say that I was mistaken and that my opinion was founded on insufficient evidence. I never saw a tumour with such big areas as Dr. Rubinstein showed me in one of these bipolar spongioblastomas with an ependymoma-like arrangement of the nuclei. In that case there was a very big area of oligodendroglioma-like tissue. Such big areas I never saw in my material. May be that I have not looked at the right sort of tumours. Thank you.

Dr. Zülch: Thank you, Dr. Ringertz.

Dr. Woolf: I believe Dr. Rubinstein is speaking again this afternoon. But he has not mentioned something which I thought provided very important support for the true origin of the tissue, that is the Mallory staining. Perhaps you can just explain why you did not mention it, before I say anything more.

Dr. Rubinstein: I did not mention Mallory staining, because having been trained with Dr. Russell, I have taken the Mallory staining for granted. Of course all these cases had PTAH staining done to establish that the cells which I showed were of glial origin. I have projected mainly van Gieson stains really from an aesthetic point of view, because they show the contrast so much better than any other stain I know.

Dr. Woolf: You will appreciate that the point I want to make is that if the neutral observer sees these two areas, he sees one area which is forming collagen, one area which does not and he wonders whether it is not all sarcomatous but that in some areas and for some reason the cells have not formed their intercellular product and I think, if we are thinking like that it is very valuable to have some definite evidence that the cells are forming glial fibres and not forming reticulin. Of course again this argument depends on accepting the fact that fibres which are stained by phosphotungstic acid-haematoxylin can only be glial fibres. That seems to be accepted quite definitely probably by the majority of people in our country anyhow. I am not sure if it is entirely accepted and I wonder whether this important point should not be worked up, so that convincing evidence is available to everyone. Probably there is not in the literature a critical trial of Mallory's stain but if there is it would be nice to be told where it is or if not perhaps someone might be encouraged to carry it out.

Dr. Zülch: I thank you, Dr. Woolf.

Dr. Rubinstein: 1 am quite willing to provide Dr. Woolf with a list of references on the Mallory stain, from the original paper of Mallory onwards. It has been used by many people particularly in the United States and in Canada from the early twenties and I think it has been well established. As regarding the evidence here I just want to add that these cases have all been studied with many stains and one striking feature is that you see with PTAH virtually the negative pciture of what you see with a van Gieson or a reticulin stain. In other words the areas which show the reticulin or the darkly staining sarcoma cells are negative with PTAH, the cells which are paler with a more cobweblike appearance are glial, do not contain reticulin, are strongly positive with PTAH and form neuroglial fibres.

Dr. Zülch: Dr. Calvo, would like to comment on this.

Dr. Calvo: I would like to say that the possibility of the sarcoma infiltrating along the blood vessels with isolated fragments of reactive brain tissue could appear as a mixed tumour, but in the cases that Dr. Rubinstein was showing us I cannot really be certain that the glial cells are reactive astrocytes, because in my opinion reactive astrocytes have a very clear vascular attachment. One of the first things that the astrocyte does when it is submitted to an inflammatory or mechanical or any other type of reaction, the first thing, that this astrocyte shows is an increase of the vascular relation. The foot plate of the expansion that goes to the blood vessels is bigger and so it emphasizes the glial-vascular relation. In the cases shown by Dr. Rubinstein I cannot distinguish any glial-vascular relation and therefore I cannot concede that the cells are reactive astrocytes surrounded by sarcomatous tissue. It looks in some of these cases as if there is glial production as derived from the neoplastic growth in the surrounding tissue and this could be responsible for the "mixed tumour" of "glial sarcomatous" type.

Dr. Zülch: Dr. Rubinstein, you want to answer?

Dr. Rubinstein: Yes, I am not entirely certain I fully understood the argument. Am I right, Dr. Calvo, in assuming that the first point you made was that you think these are just reactive astrocytes and not neoplastic ones? Is that what you . . .

Dr. Calvo: I say in many cases of sarcomatous growth the glial cells react against this growth and the sarcomatous cells growing along the blood vessels can isolate islands of brain tissue, but I think that the histological characteristic for distinguishing these reactive areas from the neoplastic ones would be the gliovascular relation which is emphasized when the glial cells are reactive, but in your cases I could not distinguish gliovascular relations at all.

Dr. Rubinstein: I get your point, Dr. Calvo. I would like to answer this, yes, that when I diagnose a glioma and I think that many people probably feel as I do, they don't pay any particular attention to the gliovascular relation. Perhaps I have been wrong about it. I took it that a malignant tissue could be recognized by characteristics like cell pleomorphism, nuclear abnormality and so forth without looking at the gliovascular structures. I have not looked in these cases particularly for this particular point and I will look again if this supports your idea.

Dr. Zülch: Thank you, Dr. Rubinstein.

Dr. Sayre: Well, I am not sure that I understand these differences of opinion. Dr. Calvo, is it true that you believe that these tumours are mixed glial tumours and sarcomas because there are no suckerfeet?

Dr. Calvo: Right.

Dr. Rubinstein: Well, I misunderstood Dr. Calvo completely then.

Dr. Calvo: Then I would like to show a case here that we could consider as one of these mixed tumours.

Dr. Zülch: Would you try to project the tumour.

Dr. Calvo: This case we treated in Brookhaven National Laboratory. The cells in the picture show the biopsy specimen stained with PTAH, there was a reticular part and a glial part. This was not considered a glioblastoma. Here you can see the spindle cells directed to the blood vessels and the walls of the tissue. The next picture was taken after the autopsy. This area shows gliosis with many giant astrocytes. We could not find any glioblastoma. The next slide, — and this was near the parietal region we found a tumour with the typical attachment to the dura mater and this was considered to be a gigantocellular sarcoma. See this enormous nucleus here, the spindle cells are of very bizarre form, some of the multinucleated resemble the foreign body cell type. Sometimes we found one nucleus and sometimes multinucleated elements with large nucleoli and occasionally some very elongated cells with two nucleoli. We can also see here some mitotic figures together with the giant cells. Now I would like to show you the reticulin formation in this occipital form of tumour. You can see practically every cell surrounded by reticulin. Both tumours were coexistent and at the operation they removed the glioblastoma but we could not find it at autopsy.

Dr. Rubinstein: Dr. Calvo, I completely accept your interpretation from your picture. I think the case is almost identical with the last case I showed in the evolution of the histological picture. You have here again the biopsy taken before and the final picture after the recurrence. Of course I don't know if your case was irradiated, it is possible that some of the giant cells may be related to irradiation but I am quite convinced by your pictures that there is a sarcoma there.

Dr. Calvo: Here is the microscopical picture with the occipital pole occupied by this hard tumour attached to the dura mater in the lower part.

Dr. Netsky: I would like also to point out that we have experimental confirmation of this in the experiments I cited. There was ostensibly a glioblastoma multiforme initially, which in successive transplants became entirely a sarcoma.

Dr. Zülch: Thank you, Dr. Netsky.

Dr. Müller: I want to ask Dr. Rubinstein, in the patient with the transformation of the glial gangliocytoma to the mixed type was there any X-ray radiation in the interval.

Dr. Rubinstein: Yes, this patient had also irradiation before her first operation, 2 courses before she was first seen in 1936 and 2 further courses, one year after operation and one after the second year.

Dr. Zülch: May I then make a few minor and perhaps some major remarks on this paper, the value of which is not at all minimized by the criticisms which I put before you because in my opinion we have to consider this problem of mixed tumours as one of the major problems of our work in the next years. May I begin with some minor remarks. First that in my opinion "palisading" would not be a sign of transformation into a glioblastoma. I have seen this palisading in focal rodlike necroses. I have seen that phenomenon of rod-like necrosis very often in oligodendrogliomas so it would only suggest to me that the growth is a little more rapid than usually. But this may be still a question of terminology. The second is the problem of the astrocytes or so-called astrocytes shown by the aniline dyes. I think even with phosphotungstic acid haematoxylin it is perhaps difficult to distinguish whether one "astrocyte-like" cell is actually of astrocytic origin or comes from the oligodendroglia side and I will show you in the next contribution a few examples of this, because even with gold sublimate, which we consider as almost specific for astrocytes and with which we actually know that the normal oligodendroglia is definitely not impregnated at all, large cells of this type are impregnated. Well, then you could say these are actually astrocytes. But they have one characteristic which as I have heard from my friend Calvo and I have always believed myself is a sign of oligodendrocytic origin. That is the clear nucleus in impregnations. When astrocytes are impregnated by gold sublimate you can never see the nucleus whereas in the oligodendrocytic giant cell in any metallic impregnation the nucleus remains clear. Am I right, Dr. Calvo?

Dr. Calvo: Yes.

Dr. Zülch: So much for the astrocytes and we may discuss this again after the paper on oligodendrogliomas.

Now I come to the major aspects of this problem. Are we not falling back a little too much into the assumption that a tumour must be "pure" with regard to cell content? Tumour growth, is by no means the growth of one cell race only. That is what we have objected to in what Bailey and his group assumed in his first book. Yet if you read his later papers, he never followed this merely cytological "puristic" aspect. And a tumour consists in the view of general pathologists of parenchyma and stroma. Well, the stroma may be very excessive. If you take a scirrhous tumour of the mammary gland you may have a few epithelial cells and a great excess of stroma which is beautifully shown in silver methods, and none of us would call this a carcinosarcoma. We must, I think, take into consideration, that even a tumour of the brain must have some stroma. This may be also excessive, and I know, and this makes clear why I am so much interested in this case, I know that Prof. Spatz when I began to work with him as a young man, always said, we have the "gliosarcoma" i. e. the glioblastoma with plenty of connective tissue and I did not like that. We had a long and hard discussion with him for years and years on this question, and I think, he still believes that there are true "gliosarcomas" which are actually mixed tumours. If we now begin to analyse the mesodermal part of the tumour, i. e. the parts of the tumour which are different from the main tumour cell, we must first of all take into consideration that we are dealing with normal tissue — I said that already yesterday — a tissue which is invaded by the tumour, and in which there are very many astrocytes which react and naturally appear in the tumour tissue. It is the same with the oligodendroglioma where there are many well preserved neurons, with axons and myelin sheaths. They probably still function because fits occur over a large number of years — even 10 to 15 years — in oligodendrogliomas. These fits must originate in a region where, if you believe in the ordinary theories of origin of fits, there are ganglion cells still acting either in the tumour itself or at least in its very close neighbourhood.

Now the second point is that some of these tumours at least are hamartomas from the very beginning i. e. have a hamartomatous dysembryogenetic origin. This certainly is true for quite a good many of the gangliocytomas. I remember the classical case in the world literature of Bielschowsky where he described for the first time a temporo-basal gangliocytoma, a tumour group which in the meantime has become very well acknowledged by the neurosurgeon and was first depicted by Schär and Christensen as a developmental tumour. Bielschowsky showed that at the moment of the invasion of the hippocampus and its neighbourhood by the mesodermal tissue which later forms the choroid plexus, a severe disturbance of the brain stroma relationship is induced and as a result a tremendous amount of mesodermal tissue is produced from the leptomeninges in which the tumour grows. I would like just to show a picture of one of these tumours. Among the mesodermal structures in this tumour islands of cells were spread which are definitely true Nissl-cells. You all know that if we get our tumours from the neurosurgeon, we are able to classify 85 to 95%. But there is a great difference between these tumours which come from neurosurgical wards and those which come from some neurological asylums where you may have severe developmental failures in the brain and where you have hamartoblastomas as in v. Recklinghausen's disease or tuberous sclerosis particularly, where you may start with a gangliocytoma and have a malignant tumour years afterwards. I would not say that this particular tumour is an integral part of tuberous sclerosis, but I could imagine that a very similar or identical tumour could occur in a patient with definite signs of tuberous sclerosis. We must not rely here too much upon the clinical features, because we have seen the specific tumours of tuberous sclerosis in the lateral ventricle with all the finer minor disturbances of the cerebral cortex in patients who were perfectly normal as regards intelligence, and had no fits and no adenoma sebaceum, so the classical triad of tuberous sclerosis was missing.

One last point I would like to stress. I mentioned the possibility of the tumours being hamartoblastomas and the need to take the regressive changes in the tumour tissue into consideration. Some of your cells look to me as if they were hydropic. Because they shrunk so much during the embedding and I could imagine that these were actually regressive parts of the tumour or tumour cells which are located in a special environment. I should mention that we noted the same — and it is this which unites us — in our classical monstrocellular sarcomas. The parts which have the monster cells usually have the smallest amount of connective tissue stroma. But I think I know from general pathology and perhaps Dr. Ringertz will be able to help us, that there are sarcomas where you have areas where the cells form an excessive amount of connective tissue and others where you have "medullary" sarcomas, i. e. sarcomas which are very cellular with only little formation of fibrils. These are only a few points which must be taken into consideration if we are to get the problem clearer and have only those cases at the end which are really convincing. These must form, I think a basic part of our discussion in one of the next meetings.

Dr. Rubinstein: I would like to take up two or three points which are rather interesting. I took pity on the members of this Symposium and tried to keep the number of slides as small as possible, but I have a reticulin picture of this ganglion cell tumour, which is identical with the picture you have shown. It is extremely interesting that in the ganglionic area you have an enormous amount of reticulin around the islands. In the glial part there is virtually no reticulin except in relation to the blood vessels. I certainly agree that in a ganglion cell tumours we have an astonishing amount of reticulin.

The second point touches the "gliosarcoma". It was Stroebe who first desribed the gliosarcomas and from his remarkable paper which is still now extremely valuable reading I am quite certain that what he regarded as gliosarcomas were truly mixed sarcomas and gliomas. It was only afterwards that the term gliosarcoma was used to include a large number of fusiform glioblastomas so that the term gliosarcoma fell into disrepute. I myself have always refused to use the term gliosarcoma because of this.

Now, concerning the first point you raised, Dr. Zülch, regarding the value of PTAH for astrocytes and the criteria of histological diagnosis. Here I must say that I do belong to the school which recognizes an astrocyte with the PTAH through its cell processes and fibres. You just emphasized the nucleus in the distinction here. Here I can really do no better than quote Prof. Zülch himself in his book, when he remarks on the nucleus that it is not the "visiting card" of the cell, that you are identifying the cell by its cytoplasmic character and not by its nucleus alone.

Dr. Zülch: Thank you so much for your remarks but I think there may be one exception which I have previously mentioned. It concerns the ganglionic cells which have a clear nucleus with a large nucleolus and thick cell membrane which are the signs of a high cellular activity. I did not mean this when I said that the lack of impregnation of the nucleus is one of the signs of the oligodendroglia. Am I right, Dr. Calvo? perhaps you comment on this, as you know, the features of the metallic methods better than any of us.

Dr. Calvo: The lack of impregnation of the nuclei in the normal oligodendroglia is one of the main features of the oligodendrocytes and I wonder if in the astrocytes it is not that a larger amount of cytoplasm is stained with the silver carbonate and this is enough to obscure the nuclei so that it appears as if these cells are filled with silver and the nuclei cannot be recognized. While in the oligodendrocytes they can be recognized because of the very small amount of cytoplasm around the nuclei. Even if the cytoplasm is quite plentiful the nuclei may lie at one pole of the cell. So although it appears to be more characteristic of oligodendrocytes to have unstained nuclei; this may not be really specific but secondary to the amount of cytoplasm surrounding the nuclei. But for practical purposes if we see a cell with a round unstained nucleus in silver carbonate preparations it can be fairly safely considered as an oligodendrocyte.

But I would emphasize much more the type of the expansions of the cells and the lack of relation of the expansions to the blood vessels as characteristic of oligodendroglias. A cell can only be considered an astrocyte, if we really see the attachment to the blood vessels which distinguishes the cell from an oligodendrocyte. But then another morphological consideration should be taken into account. The particular cells may be classified astrocytic or oligodendrocytic if we see the positive findings but not on a negative basis.

Dr. Netsky: This discussion of whether the stroma may be reactive as in the astrocytes shown by Dr. Calvo, or whether the parenchyma may be reactive is of interest to me. I should point out that all of us are using almost exclusively histologic criteria. Every expert here has confidence in his ability to distinguish malignancy, but that basic confidence may not always be justified as is shown by this discussion. I suggest that we have really to settle these problems and go beyond histologic criteria. We have to use biologic criteria, that is, growth rates in experimental animals and ultimately we might even have chemical criteria. But this dependence on histologic criteria and indeed the expression which I have heard of "histologic proof" is something that I question.

Dr. Zülch: Thank you, Dr. Netsky.

Dr. Sayre: I would just like to draw attention to the fibrosarcomas of the breast. Do we definitely have sarcomas in animals in the supportive tissue? This is well recognized and no neuropathologic material that you can have will make us believe that the tumour developed from that supporting tissue.

Dr. Zülch: That is what you can have. What I wanted to make clear is that there are pure carcinomas which they call scirrhous and where you may have 85% of stroma and 15% of parenchyma cells.

Dr. Sayre: Oh, very definitely. In the small cell carcinoma of the stomach the carcinomatous cells are only found with great difficulty there is just a mass of connective tissue with the very malignant cells in a single line. But very definitely on the other side are those well known tumours in which there is malignant growth of the connective tissue as well as the parenchymatous tissue.

Dr. Netsky: I think we can all agree on this issue of the parenchyma and the stroma, but the question I still ask is how we do know whether the stroma is reactive or cancerous.

Dr. Sayre: I ask Dr. Netsky what is the definition of cancer which was asked two days ago and I don't know whether he is really able to answer.

Dr. Netsky: I refer you to another committee!

On the Definition of the Polymorphous Oligodendroglioma

By

K. J. Zülch

Our discussion today on the oligodendroglioma is perhaps a little simpler than that on the spongioblastoma. I do not think the classical type of oligodendroglioma requires any discussion. I would like you to discuss with us today the question as to whether there is not a series of polymorphous tumours belonging to the oligodendroglioma group. In this we are following in the footsteps of *Bailey* who observed groups of polymorphous astrocyte-like cells differing from the usual honeycomb-like architecture. He was inclined to regard these cells as degenerating or transitional.

Following his observations we have been able to establish that there is a whole series of polymorphous tumours which in some parts show the classical honeycomb arrangement of the oligodendroglia while other parts show a quite atypical and severe polymorphism. In my paper in 1941 I particularly referred to this type and asked to what extent is was justifiable to include the tumours within the oligodendroglioma group. At the Neuropathological Congress in London in 1955 I again emphasized this question and pointed out that there were a great variety of deviations from the usual structure.

1. A spindle-celled part which recalled the spongioblastoma but within which it was still possible to recognize the basic honeycomb appearance.

2. A part with a certain similarity to a medullary carcinoma. We have however only infrequently encountered this type.

3. A polymorphous part with giant cells and multinucleated cells of all types, for example of the *Langhans* type thereby showing a resemblance to the glioblastoma multiforme. There are in fact described in the literature a whole series of atypical glioblastomas in whom the survival period has been unusually long and this made us think. I therefore proceeded on the working hypothesis that there is probably a polymorphous type of oligodendroglioma with the prolonged clinical history which one characteristically encounters in a normal oligodendroglioma and which has a post-operative survival period of many years, which to say the least is quite atypical for a glioblastoma. In these cases there is usually a very striking vascularisation with cellular polymorphism so that one can conclude

that the tumour has developed malignancy. This vascularisation consists particularly in the formation of larger vessels which can to some extent be demonstrated in arteriograms. Clinical experience has taught us that arteries which are visible in arteriograms and in particular those connected with veins by arteriovenous short-circuits, are evidence of a very rapid and I would say malignant growth.

We now come to the question as to whether we are actually dealing with an oligodendroglioma of classical type or a special form of a mixed astrocytic-oligodendrogliomatous tumour in which the astrocytic component has developed towards glioblastoma. We may remember at this point that *Cooper* and later *Scherer* suggested that in view of the striking intermingling of oligodendrogliomatous and astrocytic areas in certain tumours it was necessary to postulate a "mixed tumour" of the oligodendro-astrocytoma type.

The crucial evidence is provided by metallic impregnation and in this connection we have received great help from Dr. *Meller* *, a co-worker of Dr. *Calvo* who has during the last month carried out impregnations of our oligodendrogliomas in all those cases in which the oligodendrogliomatous nature of the tumour has been the object of discussion. In fact it has been possible to demonstrate — and these preparations are available to you for study — that the important part of these tumours is composed of small-celled oligodendroglia. On the other hand the large-celled portions in impregnation preparations have an external appearance which very strikingly recalls the astroblast and also many astrocytes. They even — as I already showed in 1941 — impregnate with gold sublimate; but with all impregnation methods one characteristic is present: the nucleus remains visible as a clear vacuole which is pretty characteristic for the oligodendroglia. So I believe one can actually accept the majority of these cases as constituting a malignant transformation of an oligodendroglioma. We have therefore perhaps been able at last to provide the evidence which I lacked in 1955 when *Kernohan*, who was presiding over the session, said, that whilst acknowledging my large experience in the classification of tumours he could only say that the pictures I had shown would have been diagnosed by the majority of those present in the auditorium as glioblastomas.

At the time I pointed out that at least there was no major biological difference between the isomorphic and the polymorphic types and this was of importance for the classification of *Bailey* and *Cushing*. A purely morphological classification without biological implications can have no meaning for the neurosurgeon for whom

---

* *Meller, K.*, Modifikation der Silberimprägnation zur Darstellung der Zellen des Oligodendroglioms im Paraffinmaterial. Acta neuropath. 2 (1963), 497—500.

the classification is intended. I would like to put forward today a working hypothesis for our discussion that this polymorphous oligodendroglioma is a malignant variety — that it has a higher degree of malignancy than the normal tumour.

I would be particularly greatful to Dr. *Sayre* and Dr. *Ringertz* if they would put forward their views on this concept and also if perhaps Dr. *Calvo* could contribute something through his great experience with metal impregnations. Now this is only the introduction to the discussion. We may also ask the other participants how the problem of the oligodendroglioma appears to them from their own special point of view.

Discussion

Dr. Ringertz: May I go back to the starting point of our discussion and say a few words on the diagnosis of gliomas. Naturally we have a rather frequent deviation from the so-called classical picture of the oligodendroglioma and that is why in my opinion the oligodendroglioma is very difficult to diagnose at least if you only have the so-called routine stains at your disposal. You cannot rely very much in difficult cases on the cellular picture which you obtain with ordinary stains. You have to take into consideration the vascular pattern of the tumour, the calcification and many other features. You naturally get great help from the impregnation stains, but in my opinion these are also very difficult to interpret, because there always is such a mixture of other cell types which are also shown when you impregnate these tumours. You may find astrocytes and arrangements of bipolar cells round the vessels, you may find around some vessels the picture of an astroblastoma and so on. Then we come to the polymorphism of these gliomas, the oligodendrogliomas, the signs of anaplasia of malignancy. They are naturally also very difficult to interpret just because of this admixture of other cell types. In many oligodendrogliomas which show a very monomorphous cell picture, for example, you find mitoses. This sign in my opinion is not necessarily accompanied by signs of rapid growth of a tumour. A monomorphic picture with many mitoses is not a strong indication that the tumour is growing very rapidly. On the other hand these giant cell formations may of course be a sign of malignant transformation, but I think you do see this in specimens of oligodendrogliomas which are otherwise rather uniform so that they present a rather pure oligodendrocytic picture but with an admixture of these giant cells and I am glad to hear now from Dr. Zülch that in many cases these giant cells may be identified by impregnation as really oligodendrocytic so that they are not the reaction of a mixed astroglia. When we come to these very polymorphous tumours it is naturally an interesting question whether the most polymorphous and anaplastic cells are really oligodendrocytic or if it is the astrocytic component, which is surely present in every oligodendroglioma, that grows into a glioblastoma. I have no personal opinion on that, but I was interested to see that some of Dr. Zülch's pictures here indicate that it is really the oligodendrocytic component which becomes malignant and not the astrocytic component. Thank you.

Dr. Zülch: Thank you very much, Dr. Ringertz. Would you comment, Dr. Sayre?

Dr. Sayre: This has always been a difficult question which Dr. Netsky has put forward, how do we diagnose a particular type of cell and can we be sure of it. I reviewed the histologic sections Dr. Zülch sent to us and I naturally asked Dr. Kernohan to review them also. But I am afraid that we are not able to agree with the diagnosis, to us the pictures of the polymorphous oligodendrogliomas were those which we would call ependymomas or astrocytomas of grade 3 or 4. I just would not call some of the cells oligodendrocytes which were shown in the microphotographs as oligodendrocytes, not with this particular stain at any rate. I do not have a biological report to make because not having selected the material originally I have no way of going back and saying whether there is anything in this particular group which is different. But purely on a histologic basis I am afraid I still cannot separate them. The general appearance seems to be mixed and like other individuals I am disturbed by the chart here which shows the polymorphous patients. The majority of the patients with the regular oligodendrogliomas are living and consequently their postoperativ course will be even longer than is indicated on the chart. There is a great difference between the tumours as implied by the chart alone. They do have a closer biological resemblance to the classical astrocytoma grade 3 or 4 or glioblastoma multiforme. So that whether the biological differences are quite as great as suggested is I think still open to question. So I am still basing my opinion on the general histological appearance and the biological growth as indicated. They are not really the same tumour.

Dr. Zülch: For support I can only call upon Dr. Calvo who has seen all the impregnations and he is of the opinion that these tumours are actually of oligodendrocytic origin. I join you in your opinion that these are malignant oligodendrogliomas ·and I would, grade them, in my classification one step lower i. e. grade III. But quite a good many of those patients are still surviving, 2, 3 years which is not the usual survival period for glioblastomas. The majority of the patients with fusiform glioblastomas die at the end of the first year. Grade 2 would best include perhaps the normal oligodendrogliomas and grade 3 this particular form.

Dr. Sayre: I would agree that when an oligodendroglioma becomes considerably dedifferentiated it may be we are not capable of separating it from the standard astrocytoma and that the group glioblastoma multiforme does include perhaps groups of tumours that we can't separate one from the other. This again, Dr. Netsky, I think, has suggested from his studies. But at the moment I don't have sufficient information to say that they are malignant oligodendrogliomas. Neither in my review nor in Dr. Kernohan's review could we substantiate the conclusion that they were oligodendrogliomas. To us they looked like malignant ependymomas and malignant astrocytomas.

Dr. Zülch: Thank you very much, Dr. Sayre. Would you comment, Dr. Calvo.

Dr. Calvo: I would like to show a few slides of our case AO which was a woman of 35 years of age. The tumour was located in the frontal lobe on both sides and had preoperative symptoms of 4 months with a survival time of 2 years. The first slide shows the extension of the tumour in a brain section including the corpus callosum of the opposite hemisphere. And this is a myelin stain of the brain sections. Now I would like to show you the tumour with various silver impregnations.

I think you see the homogeneity of the cells with a round nucleus a typical example of an oligodendrocytic architecture.

Dr. Netsky: Are some of these cells in ependymal rosettes or how you interpret them?

Dr. Calvo: I don't think so. It looks as though there has been a retraction of the tissue in paraffin, but the nuclei are very close to the capillaries and they do not have the thin perivascular expansions of the ependymoma. In the next slide you see some areas in which the round type of oligodendrocyte is observed but there is a giant astrocyte at the periphery of the tumour. One of the problems is to decide whether these cells are reactive astrocytes or whether they are components of an astrocytic type of oligodendroglioma. You know that Hortega in his time already admitted that he regarded many oligo-dendrogliomas as really a mixture of oligodendrocytes and astrocytes in blasto-matous proliferation, therefore he diagnosed many cases as oligodendro-astro-cytomas. I will show you many areas with giant astrocytes and intermixed with these cells there are still oligodendrocytes, but on the other hand there are pure proliferations of oligodendrocytes. Now with this haematoxylin and eosin section it would be difficult to decide if this is a polymorphous oligo-dendrocytoma with a bizarre type of cell or whether these cells are astrocytes. This section was stained with a variant of Hortega's reticulin technique and you can see the reticulin formation on the blood vessels producing this sort of semi-lobulation in the tumour which has some similarity to the ependy-momas. This proliferation of the blood vessels is very characteristic of what we may call the oligodendroblastoma. The network of blood vessels is very dense, but it is interesting to note .the absence of the expansions which one would expect in an ependymoma. The cells are very close to the capillaries and all of them have these round nuclei with very narrow cytoplasm around the nuclei giving this honeycomb appearance of the oligodendrocytic tissue. In another of Hortega's impregnations you notice that some of these cells are clearly astrocytes. Altogether it is a quite uniform appearance in the tumour although it is true that not all the cells are stained as I pointed out previously. I have to remind you that not all oligodendrocytes of neoplastic nature are impregnated with silver.

Dr. Zülch: And there in the middle and left upper corner of your slide I saw plenty of oligodendrocytes.

Dr. Calvo: Plenty with a clear nucleus and very few expansions which never go to the blood vessels.

Dr. Zülch: Yes, and I repeat there were some astrocytes as in my metallic impregnation too. There is no doubt about that.

Dr. Calvo: But we don't see this perivascular arrangement typical of astro-cytomas. The cells and expansions are visible all round but I don't see here any clear relation to the blood vessel. Here is a clear nucleus but only one expansion, the cytoplasm is polarized, on one side there is the nucleus and on the other the cytoplasm. There are very few expansions, sometimes screw formation and the absence of vascular relation and this, I think, is character-istic of this type of cells. In others these expansions may be splitting into two or three. But I would like to show you another anilin stain in order to find some other morphological features of the cells. Now we see in colour what we saw before in black and white. Sometimes we have a proliferation of the blood vessels in the region of the tumour. A higher magnification shows these blood vessels without any relation to the tumour cells at all. They lie very close to the blood vessels but they never show any expansions that go to the blood vessels as a vascular foot as a "sucker foot". Now if we see occasional cells that have this definite relation to the blood vessels I think they may correspond to astrocytes in the invaded brain tissue. But never do we see many cells with a relation to the blood vessels. Next slide please. One of the characteristics of this stain is the difference in the staining ability of the nuclei. The nucleus is pyknotic though you still can see the very small amount of cytoplasm with the nucleus on one side, the ctyoplasm on the other and a few expansions can be distinguished. In a younger cell we see bigger expansions and in another a larger amount of cytoplasm, but never a relation of these cells to the vessels. Another type of stain, shows the nuclei very well including mitotic division and in other parts several different stages of this can be seen. Another PAN stain from the same but this is taken from to an astrocytoma. We find very large cells with green cytoplasm, the nuclei are oval shaped and these cells show clear relations with the blood vessels.

Dr. Rubinstein: Dr. Calvo, may I just ask how do you interpret the bigger cells?

Dr. Calvo: These were astrocytes with a clear relation of the expansions to the wall of the blood vessels.

Dr. Ringertz: Do you classify this as an astrocytoma? With so many oligocytes?

Dr. Calvo: Most of the cells of the tumour send these expansions, producing a sort of sheath around the capillary before ending with foot plates. The whole tumour is filled with this sort of prolongations.

Dr. Zülch: Could it not be one of those tumours in which large parts of surrounding tissue are invaded at one of the edges and where the astrocytes show a progressive reaction and increase in number because they are invaded only by a minority of oligodendroglia cells. Dr. Ringertz and myself had the same feeling that we are not quite sure that this was not the edge of an oligodendroglioma with a marked macrogliosis at the edge.

Dr. Zülch: Would you like to comment first, Dr. Sayre.

Dr. Sayre: I just want to make sure in my own mind what Dr. Calvo's diagnosis was on this case. My own diagnosis was a mixed tumour both of oligodendroglioma and astrocytoma. I would like to know whether his opinion was that this was a pure oligodendroglioma.

Dr. Calvo: I have shown the silver impregnation. One area showed astrocytes and we have to consider whether they are reactive astrocytes at the margin between and normal brain tissue or an astrocytoma. This is very interesting and could be discussed with the mixed tumours of Dr. Rubinstein. I think it would be very important if we can decide how to know if a given cell should be considered as reactive or neoplastic and I think that what Dr. Netsky pointed out brings us to the kind of logic dominating bacteriology. The bacteriologists never admit that the stain is enough to say that this is such or such a microbe, they have to have cultures, and then they need to prove that the microbe produced a disease and only then are they sure that it is a pneumococcus or Koch's bacillus.

Dr. Zülch: Thank you. Dr. Netsky?

Dr. Netsky: We must all heartily agree on that. We should limit ourselves on these histologic criteria. What you do, and we should understand the deficiencies, is use stains to determine the criteria for recognition of normal cells and then apply them to abnormal neoplastic cells. We are not sure the same rules apply.

Dr. Zülch: You did the same for the phosphotungstic acid, because you said you can easily distinguish glial and mesodermal fibres in a tumour by phosphotungstic acid haematoxylin and this is a criterion similar to those used by Dr. Calvo.

Dr. Netsky: This is an assumption which we have not proved yet. We all accept it, but the question is, is it true? What we are attempting to say is that these cells derive from oligocytes. We have a static slide, we do not see the transition of one cell into another and until we see the actual transition we may be wrong in saying this cell looks like this and this like this, therefore a line has been established. Finally you are seeing in the silver stains and the gold stains only a fragment of the cell, as you know from electron microscopy, so you are passing an opinion on a large cell on some minor details. I submit that these considerations should make us very cautious in deciding whether this is an astrocyte or an oligodendrocyte and indeed if there is any difference between them, because they may be interchangeable.

Dr. Zülch: Thank you, Dr. Netsky.

Dr. Müller: In the last year I was at the European Anatomic Congress at Strasbourg and there was a report on the normal glia and it was pointed out that it is not possible to be certain that oligodendroglia cells can change into astrocytes in normal brain tissue. I think it is even more difficult to decide for a neoplasm.

Dr. Zülch: Thank you, Dr. Müller. I think there is a parallel in the connective tissues. Any connective tissue cell may either develop into a chondroplast or an osteoplast or lipoplast or anything else as we see beautifully in the meningiomas where you have osteoplastic, chondroplastic and lipoplastic parts as well as fibroplastic or myxoplastic. So this is an absolute parallel and one day it may be proved for the brain that cells can change if not in the mature stage at least in the immature or indifferentiated stage, when the tumour begins to grow. Dr. Rubinstein wants to speak.

Dr. Rubinstein: I am somewhat less anxious than Dr. Netsky on this question of techniques and more inclined to accept Dr. Calvo's interpretation of the tumours he has projected. I can agree with him that what he has shown us astrocytes are astrocytes and what he shows as oligodendroglia are oligodendrocytes in the silver technique he has used. I am also quite convinced that many of the pictures he has shown with other stains are of what I would recognize as oligodendrogliomas, but now we come to the pleomorphic tumours that Dr. Zülch has shown and here I think the question becomes much more difficult. I agree with Dr. Ringertz, that once you have a very pleomorphic and anaplastic tumour the difficulties in diagnosis on the basis of an identification of cells increase greatly. Now I can mainly judge from the cases which were sent to me from this laboratory and from the tissue which I examined using paraffin sections with HE and Mallory's PTAH. In the majority of cases I would never for a moment have imagined that they could be oligodendrogliomas, although I tried to persuade myself that perhaps they could be. In this I support Dr. Sayre in his feeling that the majority of these cases should be interpreted as either malignant astocytoma or just glioblastomas.

Dr. Zülch: May I ask you in the mean time, have you seen the oligodendroglia impregnations we have prepared?

Dr. Rubinstein: I have not seen these preparations. I can judge only on what I have seen. But I foresee some difficulties in accepting on the usual technique this concept of the pleomorphic oligodendroglioma. And I really find it difficult to improve on Dr. Kernohan's statement in 1955, that if this cases were shown to a large member of people the majority would not recognize the oligodendrogliomatous component. I don't think I would myself, nor would I frankly expect anyone else to do so.

Dr. Zülch: Thank you, Dr. Rubinstein.

Dr. Luginbühl: I am not trying to steal the lime-light from the polymorphous oligodendrogliomas. As I am on the program I would like to draw attention to some other features or observations I made in animal oligodendrogliomas.

Oligodendrogliomas in Animals***

By

H. Luginbühl

With 7 Figures

My contribution on the theme of oligodendrogliomas is based on 35 tumours spontaneously occuring in animals. The bovine species and the mouse account for one case each, whereas 33 were observed in dogs. The following demonstrations are based on these 33 cases.

Breed distribution:

The brachycephalic breeds account for 27 cases (82%), i. e. 23 Boxers, 2 Boston Terriers and 2 Bulldogs. Only a few cases were observed in other breeds and therefore, despite the heterogenicity in this group, we can assume a definite disposition on the part of brachycephalic breeds to the incidence of oligodendrogliomas. Various authors have already remarked on this predisposition. We can confirm their observations and add that the majority of gliomas belong to the group of oligodendrogliomas. The reason for this correlation is still unknown; a possible dysontogenetic origin for this type of neoplasm will be discussed in later publications.

Age of morbidity:

Except for 3 cases, the age of morbidity lies between 5 and 11 years, comprising therefore the middle aged and elderly animals corresponding to the middle and later decades in man. Upon appearance of the first symptoms, many of the animals were killed for humane reasons. It was difficult to determine either the time interval between the recognition of clinical symptoms and the time of death, or the average duration of the illness, because of the relatively limited number of cases and the impossibility of assessing

* This study was supported by Grant B 1916 of the National Institute for Nervous Diseases and Blindness, Bethesda 14, Maryland, USA. and Swiss Nat. Foundation for Scientific Research.

** This paper is dedicated to Prof. Dr. *K. J. Zülch,* Director of the Max-Planck-Institute for Brain Research, Cologne-Merheim. for his continuous help and encouragement.

the symptomatology from the subjective point of view. Apparently the average course of illness is much shorter than in man and many range from several days to a few months.

Sex distribution:

Out of 31 dogs of known sex, 22 (71%) were males, and 9 (29%) females. We must add that as a whole our material consists of more males than females, since more males than females are generally kept as pets.

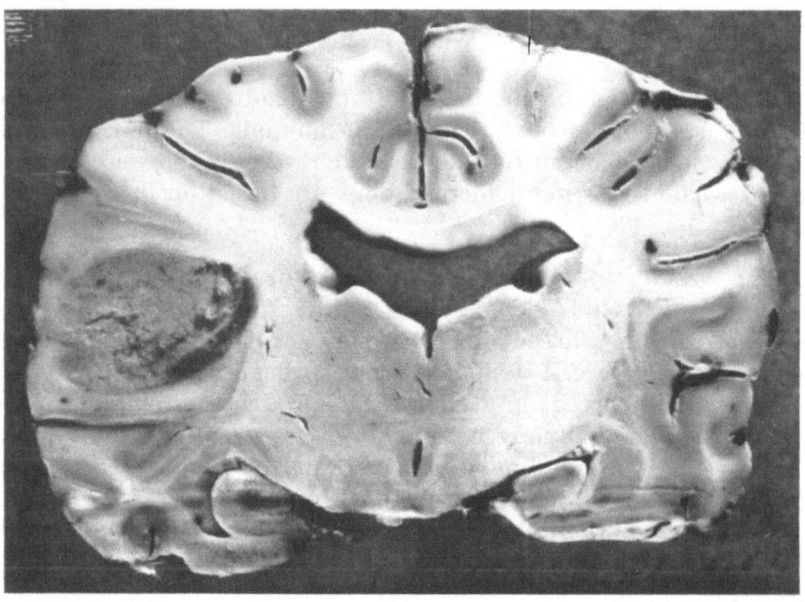

Fig. 1. Oligodendroglioma, left temporal lobe (4179); Boxer, 5 years old, male. The well defined glioma apparently grows from the central white matter, has reached the surface and infiltrates the leptomeninx. Cystic change can be seen in the deep part of the tumour. Moderate hydrocephalus lacking interventricular septum as often seen in brachycephalic breeds. Case submitted by Dr. *T. C. Jones*, Angell Memorial Animal Hospital, Boston.

Localisation:

In one case the material did not permit accurate localisation. In the other 32 cases, the gross anatomical site was as follows: frontal and olfactory lobes: 12 cases, temporal lobe and area piriformis: 8, brainstem: 8, occipital and parietal lobes: 4. In 18 cases (56%) the tumour either was contiguous to the ventricle, or had transgressed the ependyma (Figs. 2 and 4). In 3 cases it was located in the interventricular septum. The remainder were apparently growing from the depth of the centrum ovale (Fig. 1).

Macroscopic appearance:

Oligodendrogliomas usually show considerable size and extension when animals either are sacrificed or die. Only rarely are single convolutions affected and greatly expanded. The tumour thus infiltrates the cortex, reaching its surface and can raise it. In most cases, the tumour appears macroscopically well defined from the adjacent brain. There are also areas which merge imperceptibly with the normal brain, thus indicating an infiltrating mode of

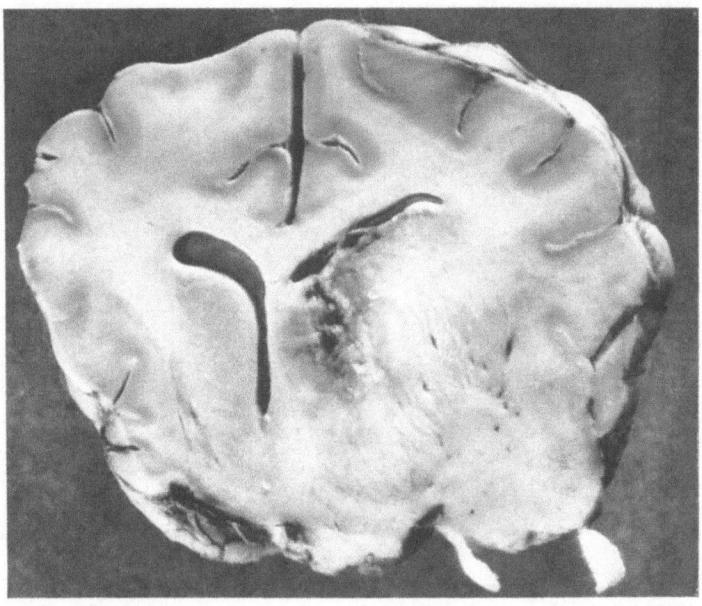

Fig. 2. Oligodendroglioma contiguous to and within right lateral ventricle and interventricular septum (4181); Boston Terrier, 11 years old, female. The glioma is ill defined and morphologically shows a rapid and infiltrative mode of growth. Note the displacement of the midline to the left. Case submitted by Dr. *T. C. Jones*, Angell Memorial Animal Hospital, Boston.

growth (Fig. 2). The unfixed tumour tissue is greyish to pinkish red. Haemorrhages are frequent. Typical oligodendrogliomas have a soft consistency. This, however, shows appreciable variations, depending on regressive changes and mesenchymatous proliferations (Figs. 3 and 4).

Microscopic appearance:

We observe in the majority of cases, at least in parts, the honeycombed structure and nuclear forms found in human oligodendrogliomas (Fig. 3). In the zone infiltration, the nuclei have a tendency

to arrange themselves in rows, semi-circles and rosette-like structures. They can also deviate from their usual circular and uniform
appearance and appear elongated, rodshaped and sickle-shaped.
Mitoses are rare, but occasionally are present. In some instances a
tumour presents a disorderly architecture with considerable nuclear
polymorphism, which indicates, in our opinion, a malignant evolution. The oligodendrogliomas grow by infiltration and destroy
the pre-existing tissue, although quite deep in the tumour one may

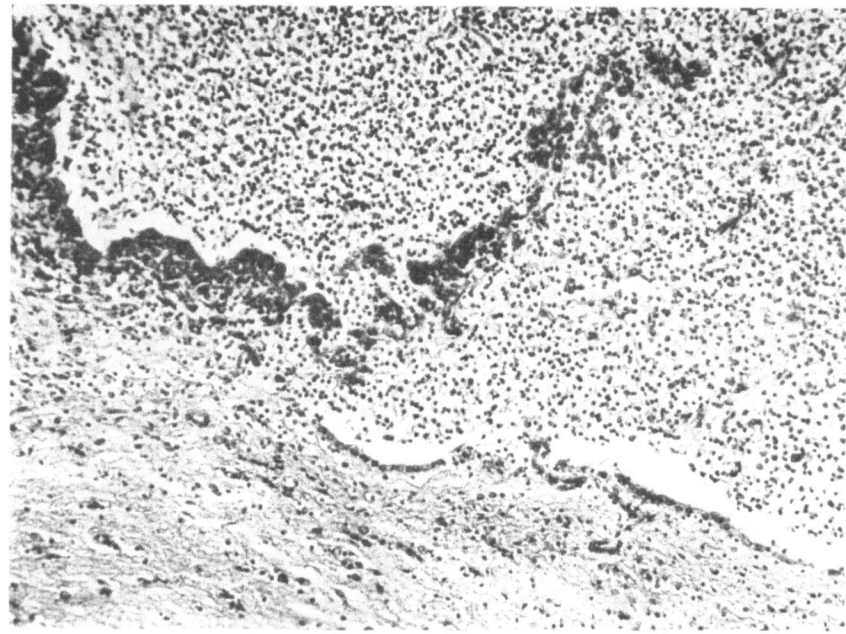

Fig. 3. Oligodendroglioma (4175); Boxer, 5 years old, male. Intraventricular growth. Honeycombed appearance, wall formed by proliferated capillaries. Note normal ependyma. Van
Gieson 144 ×. Case submitted by Dr. T. C. Jones, Angell Memorial Animal Hospital, Boston

observe an occasional pre-existing structure which may apparently
survive for a considerable time. Occasional unquestionable oligodendrogliomas grow not only along a broad front in the usual zone
of infiltration, but also along the blood vessels. Perivascular cellular
collections may be observed a few millimeters away from the gross
margin of the tumour.

Vascularity and capillary proliferation:

The vessels which are present in moderate density are, in some
areas at least, thin-walled, dilated like sinusoids, and have a

tendency to spontaneous haemorrhage. More than in other gliomas in animals, the capillaries in oligodendrogliomas proliferate to form dense and broad barriers, loops, and glomerular formations (Figs. 3 and 4). These may border zones of mucinous degeneration or be present in the absence of regressive changes, and may represent an attempt to wall off the tumour from the adjacent brain tissue. In addition, considerable capillary proliferations penetrate the tumour tissue in disorderly fashion in such number that in some

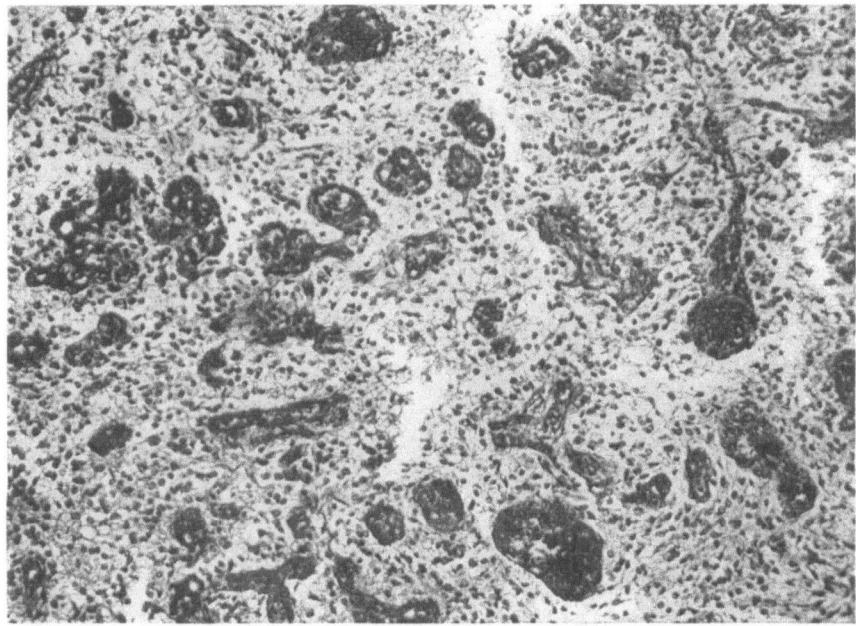

Fig. 4. Oligodendroglioma left frontal lobe (3513); Shepherd dog, 9 years old, female. Extensive capillary proliferations (loops and glomerular formations). Case submitted by Drs. E. *Dahme* and B. *Schiefer*, Munich.

areas they surpass in cell numbers and density the gliomatous tumourous component. It is therefore hardly surprising that occasionally oligodendrogliomas with a strong mesodermal element have been regarded as haemangioendotheliomas by those who have submitted them to us.

Regressive changes:

The most important regressive changes are mucinous and cystic degeneration. True necroses are rare and fatty changes were observed only in single isolated cells. In contrast to human tumours, oligodendrogliomas in animals lack any extensive calcifications. In some cases an occasional small calcospherite was found but never to such extent that any could be demonstrated radiologically.

Satellitosis:

These are observed in a few cases and only in occasional areas.

Round cell infiltration:

In many examples of brain tumours observed in dogs, including

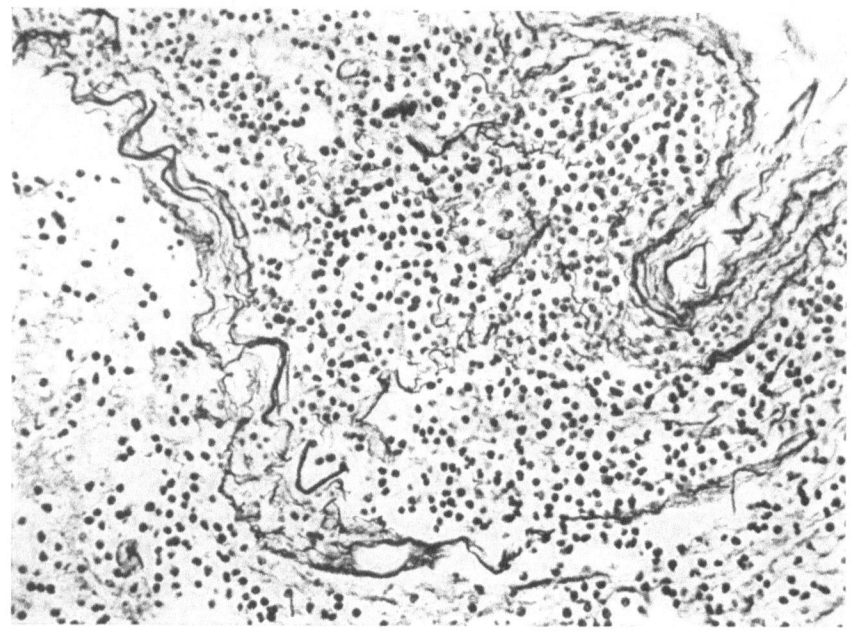

Fig. 5. Oligodendroglioma right temporal lobe (4182); Boxer, 10 years old, male. Leptomeninx infiltrated with tumour cells. Note honeycombed structure. Gomori silver impregnation (Reticulin), 300 ×. Case submitted by Dr. *T. C. Jones*, Angell Memorial Animal Hospital, Boston.

oligodendrogliomas, cellular collections can be demonstrated in the tumour tissue and its environs, but such are rarely independent of the blood vessels. These cells have the morphological features of lymphoid elements.

Relationship to leptomeninges and metastases:

As in man, many oligodendrogliomas in dogs grow from the depth toward the brain surface (Fig. 1) and tend to infiltrate the leptomeninges (Fig. 5). Among others, the cell masses grow as superficial formations in the outer cortical layers, thus presenting subpial

zones of growth. The tumour portions which grow into the leptomeninges fill the arachnoidal meshwork and may present a definitely altered architecture. In general, only a circumscribed area
of the leptomeninges is infiltrated, although extensive meningeal
cellular infiltrations were also observed in a few cases (Figs. 6 and
7). In several oligodendrogliomas adjacent to the ventricle, metastases via the cerebrospinal fluid pathway had taken place, which
in 3 cases led to generalised seeding throughout the ventricular
system and the meninges (Fig. 6 and 7).

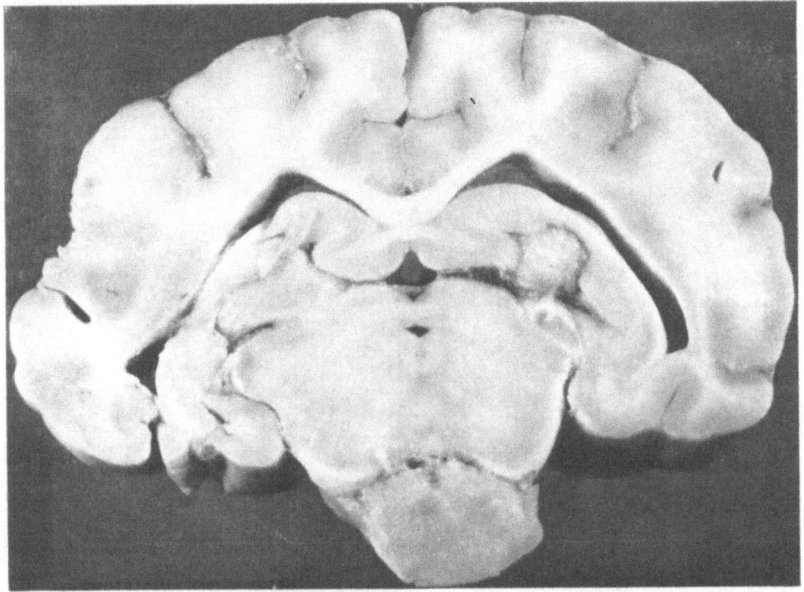

Fig. 6. Oligodendroglioma, diencephalon adjacent to third ventricle with meningeal infiltration
in infundibular region (3139); Boxer, 10 years old, male. Large tumour masses in leptomeninx
(base of brain and hippocampus).

Differential diagnoses:

A few oligodendrogliomas are difficult to distinguish by their
location, architecture and cell form from ependymomas and small-
cell glioblastomas. As far as our present observations permit, we
believe that the strong mesodermal component is a special characteristic of oligodendrogliomas in dogs. This distinction, however, is
a matter of degree only. The association of zones with a strong
mesodermal element, of honeycomb architecture, of oligodendroglioma-like nuclei, and of typical regressive changes, raises a

12*

strong suspicion of oligodendroglioma. A possible confusion with neoplasms of capillary origin is worthy of note.

Acknowledgement:

This study was made possible through the contribution of cases by the following members of the Commission for Comparative Neuropathology (WFN):

Dr. *T. C. Jones,* Angell Memorial Animal Hospital, Boston,

Prof. *S. van den Akker,* Faculty of Vet. Med., University of Utrecht,

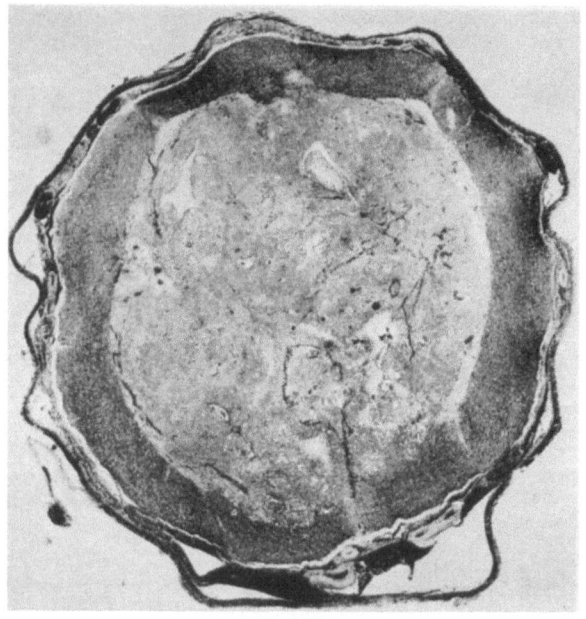

Fig. 7. Oligodendroglioma, occipital lobe adjacent to lateral ventricle; generalized seeding throughout the ventricular system and the meninges (3772); Boxer, $6^{1}/_{2}$ years old, male. "Stiftgliom" growing in cervical cord. Note tumour cells in leptomeninx. Luxol fast blue Cresyl, low power magnification. Case submitted by Prof. *S. van den Akker,* Utrecht.

Drs. *E. Dahme* and *B. Schiefer,* Vet. Path. Dept., University of Munich,

Dr. *J. B. M. Gellatly,* Royal Dick School of Vet. Studies, University of Edinburgh,

Prof. *G. Pallaske,* Vet. Path. Institute, University of Gießen,

Prof. *H. Stünzi,* Vet. Path. Institute, University of Zürich.

The author and Prof. Dr. *E. Frauchiger,* Secretary of the Commission, wish to thank the contributors for their valuable assistance.

Discussion

Dr. Zülch: Thank you, Dr. Luginbühl. But I see you have still some remarks to make.

Dr. Luginbühl: As I pointed out, the bulk of these tumours were adjacent to the lateral ventricle and even encroaching upon it as one can see in a section of a frontal lobe with a large tumour filling up the lateral ventricle. This is a very interesting and typical localisation in the majority of cases, but sometimes at the level of the anterior commissure the tumour seems to have begun to invade the interventricular septum. It may be of considerable size and grows in both directions into the lateral fields of large parts of the 3rd ventricle. Macroscopically and sometimes even microscopically these tumours can hardly be differentiated from those we usually consider as ependymomas. In another case also the gyri are affected with extension of the tumour to the surface and the meninges. There we have just a small part of it and it is away from the main part of the tumour but we have considerable subpial growth of the same type of cell. I don't know whether this is a type of induction or whether the tumour has grown through both layers of meninges. Another interesting feature is a subependymal capillary proliferation which can be observed at some distance from the main tumour and we even see a growth along vessels. The architecture is somewhat changed, but if you look at other sections it will be clearly shown that this is actually an oligodendroglioma. I wonder whether this tendency to glomerular formations, even to hemorrhages is different from what you usually see in human oligodendrogliomas, I wonder whether this tumour of dogs does not show some of the characteristics of the human glioblastoma. In some cases the vascular component was so prominent that they were called haemangioendotheliomas or other vascular tumours. Next the typical features of oligodendroglioma i. e. satellitosis was seen in a few cases and also round cell infiltration. Remarkable was the high incidence of "lymphoid" infiltration around capillaries, in the meninges and so on, which is also very often seen in human oligodendrogliomas. We also observed spontaneous spread as in the infundibular recess of the 3rd ventricle and other parts, for instance in the meninges, all around the midbrain. In one case we saw something like a track glioma in the cervical cord. A large part of the cord was replaced by this typical tumour tissue with infiltration of the meninges at the same time.

Dr. Zülch: Thank you, Dr. Luginbühl, for this beautiful demonstration of the tumours in animals and again it may be worthwhile to discuss some features of this. I think a comparative neuropathology of animal and human tumours will be a very valuable task for the future and we are very grateful for this glimpse of animal pathology, with which most of us are not familiar. Does anybody want to comment?

Dr. Sayre: These are very beautiful pictures, and very beautiful demonstrations and I would not have any hesitation in agreeing that these tumours are oligodendrogliomas. It is perfectly true that there are differences between animal tissue and human tissue. I sometimes get quite lost in diagnosing reactive tissue in animals and infarcts and things like that, but certainly if the usual criteria are used these were oligodendrogliomas and it is very interesting that they should occur ...

Dr. Luginbühl: I would just like to emphasize that these studies are still at the very beginning; two years ago we had only a very few cases. Now I have almost 400 as a result of the many contributions of colleagues. I am sure within 2 or 3 years I will have a thousand cases and then I can probably say more because you all deal with series of thousands of human cases and we must first establish the kind of basis which was established 20 years or more ago in human neuropathology.

Dr. Zülch: I think we all admire your resourcefulness in tracking down these cases. Thank you very much, Dr. Luginbühl.

Dr. Netsky: Is the higher incidence of inflammation in the perivascular regions in these brain tumours related to the higher incidence of meningo-encephalitis in dogs, as opposed to man?

Dr. Zülch: May I ask if it is a definite sign of inflammation if you see "lymphoid" cells in the neighbourhood of a tumour, because they may be undeveloped tumour cells as for example in the pinealoma where it seems to be established that large epithelial cells can develop from these lymphoid cells. We see the same in gangliocytomas where some of these lymphoid cells are called neuroblasts and it is thought that they develop in the brain from ganglionic elements, so it may be reasonable that these are immature cells in an oligodendroglioma.

Dr. Netsky: Yes, this is the same problem. We still have difficulty in distinguishing neoplastic from other types of cell, I merely wanted to know whether there was a high incidence of meningo-encephalitis in these animals and whether this bore any relation to the cellular accumulation whatever the nature of the cell.

Dr. Luginbühl: There is no relation to a higher incidence of inflammation. I think, we would have to talk all night if we want to take into the discussion the encephalitides of dogs which I have frequently seen. But I am sure in these cases there is no direct relation.

Dr. Sayre: I would only like to add that the presence of lymphocytes does not necessarily require an infectious aetiology. Any general condition may call out the lymphocytes and I would not be surprised at lymphocytic tumours.

Dr. Zülch: "Symptomatic" inflammation in the sense of Spielmeyer. Dr. Calvo wants to comment.

Dr. Calvo: I would like to show a slide of our case stained for blood vessels, with the method of Biondi, a variation of the gold sublimate of Cajal using calcium permanganate. Now you see exactly the same picture as Dr. Luginbühl has just shown: glomerulus formation of blood vessels and also a very thin network of small capillaries. I think this is interesting from the histological point of view because if we don't have blood inside the capillary we cannot visualize the vessels with the other methods, but only with the Biondi stain.

Dr. Calvo: In a higher magnification we recognize how thin these capillaries are and you may even wonder if endothelial cells could be there. But these blood vessels have a very small amount of reticulin in the capillaries or venules. In no other tumour could I see a network of capillaries as dense as in this type of tumour that we consider as an oligodendroblastoma.

Dr. Zülch: Thank you, Dr. Calvo. I know that Dr. Brucher has wanted to tell us something already for a long time. May I ask him now to comment?

Dr. Brucher: I should like to show you a few slides of this curious and provoking case of polymorphous oligodendroglioma and I will draw your attention to the particular feature which seems to be important.

Dr. Zülch: Dr. Sayre, what is your diagnosis of this, if you see it at the first sight?

Dr. Sayre: Oligodendroglioma.

Dr. Zülch: Yes, in spite of the left upper corner?

Dr. Sayre: In spite of it. Oligodendrogliomas may have giant cells.

Dr. Zülch: Yes, the slides which I have sent to all of you have long and broad areas of this and they have polymorphous fields as well.

Dr. Sayre: I was not able to find that particular type of change.

Dr. Brucher: Yes, here you see a little giant cell and here a big one, and there is the Langhans arrangement of the nuclei. But you also see the honeycomb appearance and more giant cells with very dark nuclei in the Langhans disposition. In another corner one finds the Langhans type with many filaments. It is not pathognomic of the polymorphous oligodendrogliomas but I think that it is very frequently seen in these cases.

Dr. Sayre: I would agree that the first slide was an oligodendroglioma, the second slide I would agree is possibly one grade beyond that. The third stands in between, the number of oligocytes decreases and the number of astrocytic and giant forms increases.

Dr. Zülch: I think this correct if we take a classical view. There may however be a malignant transformation in an oligodendroglioma. If we persuade you that these large cells have still definite signs of oligodendrogliocytic origin what are we going to say then, how are we going to label those tumours?

Dr. Sayre: I cannot from my own experience make a judgement on them today. This particular type of Langhans giant cell is one that I am not familiar with.

Dr. Zülch: Now I would not say that this Langhans type of cell is the only type of polymorphous transformation in these tumours but since we have been searching for them we meet them very often and I often feel in a very difficult position because the number of oligodendrogliomas in our collection may then be far too high at least higher than in most of the other collections. I feel relieved by the knowledge that the Mayo figure is very high too as compared with Bailey's original figure of 2% of the intracranial tumours and he probably abided by a very strict definition for the oligodendroglioma. But this discussion on the definition of the polymorphous oligodendroglioma still remains open. What we want in this Symposium is just to emphasize the problems which everybody may face in his daily work and if we meet again some years later we will be perhaps in a better position to solve these questions.

Dr. Sayre: Yes, I was perhaps overstating and not exactly correctly interpreting your question earlier, I agree with you about this being an oligodendroglioma. The other cases which you sent us were considered to be astrocytomas with the exception of one case, that was according to you an ependymoma and I thought it was an astrocytoma.

Dr. Zülch: Thank you. Dr. Rubinstein?

Dr. Rubinstein: I just want to add to Dr. Sayre's remarks about the specific diagnoses on the slides that you sent to us. I did not know what Dr. Sayre's opinion was until to-day now and I just see from my own notes, that my diagnoses correspond exactly with his including the two that he accepts and the others he did not accept.

Dr. Zülch: Perhaps it would be a good thing if we have enough material to get Dr. Meller to make good oligodendroglia impregnations and send to all of you. Another proposition would be, to establish a collection of odd questionable cases. I suggest to exchange in the next years also cases which are either very typical spongioblastomas of the Dorothy Russell definition and not accepted by the other ones to be spongioblastomas, or are spongioblastomas

12a*

on a different terminology. To locate these in one place where they are available to everybody who wants to see them and to study them, thus providing a material stained with every informative method to help solve the problems of terminology. I think we may end the forenoon session if you have not any particular comments to make. I just want to thank Dr. Calvo for his contribution. I think at least that some of us may have learnt from Dr Calvo, that perhaps we have underestimated a little bit the metallic work of the Spanish school for some time. The session is closed, thank you Gentlemen!

V. Sarcoma and Related Processes

Dr. Zülch: I open the session on the "Sarcomas of the brain" and related processes, where Drs. Bingas, Brucher, Rubinstein and myself will give short introductions.

Primary Sarcomas of the Brain

By

K. J. Zülch

The primary sarcomas of the brain have up to now belonged to a poorly demarcated and defined group of intracranial tumours. Of course it is now a long time since a whole series of tumours were incorrectly designated as "sarcomas" — oligodendrogliomas, medulloblastomas, meningiomas — this can in part be traced back to Virchow's definition. It is no longer permissable to use the sarcoma as a dumping ground for otherwise unclassifiable tumours. In general pathology very clear definitions of sarcomas are now available for our guidance.

Amongst the malignant mesodermal tumours occuring within the cranial cavity are various types which fulfill the definition of sarcoma. Different authors such as *Hsu* and *Abbott* and *Kernohan* and *Cushing* have concerned themselves with this question. I have in a report [*] arranged the groups in the literature in the following way:

1. Diffuse sarcomatosis of the meninges, or diffuse meningeal sarcoma.

2. Diffuse sarcomatosis of the vessels, or periadventitial sarcoma.

3. So-called sarcoma of the cerebellum.

4. So-called monstrocellular sarcoma.

5. Fibrosarcoma of the dura mater.

6. Primary reticulo-sarcoma of the brain, in which one may experience difficulty in the differential diagnosis, since as we shall see — and as *Wilke* for the first time clearly demonstrated — there are all intermediate stages up to the formation of reticular-histiocytic granulomatous encephalitis. This should be an important talking point in our discussion. I will suggest that we should first try to agree on the definition of these 6 groups, in order that those which are really important may be discussed in detail. To this end perhaps Dr. *Bingas* can give us quickly a short survey of the types.

---

[*] *Zülch, K. J.,* and *B. Bingas,* Revista Brasileira de Cirurgia 45 (1963), 234 to 245: Sôbre os Sarcomas Primitivos do Cerebro.

On the Primary Sarcomas of the Brain

By

B. Bingas

In *Zülch's* classification of 6000 brain tumours (1957*) there were 162 cases of sarcoma, i. e. 2.7%. 130 of these cases were accepted for more detailed classification, since adequate material was present. They could be classified within the above mentioned group as follows:

1. Diffuse sarcoma of the meninges 9.
2. Diffuse sarcomatosis of the vessels (adventitial sarcoma) 4.
3. Sarcoma of the cerebellum 5.
4. Circumscribed sarcoma of the vessels: monstrocellular sarcoma 79.
5. Fibrosarcoma of the dura mater 30.
6. Retothelsarcoma (Reticulosarcoma) 6.

1. *Diffuse sarcomatosis of the meninges (diffuse meningeal sarcomatosis):* Unequivocal cases were reported in particular by *Connor* and *Cushing* who like *Zülch* (1956)** described the leptomeninges as cloudy resembling a leptomeningitis, the large cisterns often being permeated by plaque like tumour infiltration which surrounds the structures such as arteries and nerves which are passing through them. On the other hand, and especially at the base of the brain and in the cerebellum nut-sized tumours may be found. The histological appearances are very characteristic. A diffuse aggregation of partly lymphocytic and partly longer or spindle shaped cells with hyperchromatic nuclei are found in the leptomeninges. Numerous mitoses and extension of cells along the perivascular spaces and the cerebral cortex are very characteristic. Of our 9 cases, 5 were male and 4 female. All age groups were equally affected. The youngest patient was 2, the eldest 61 years. The prognosis must be considered highly malignant and very little better than that of the medulloblastoma.

---

* *Zülch, K. J.,* Brain Tumours. Springer-Publ. Comp., New York, 1957.

** *Zülch, K. J.,* Handb. d. Neurochir., Bd. III, 1—702, Springer-Verlag, Berlin-Göttingen-Heidelberg, 1956.

2. *Diffuse sarcomatosis of the vessels:* Adventitial sarcoma. The first case, extensively described by *Környey* was in accordance with our findings. It was certainly necessary to make sure that one was not dealing with a metastatic blastomatosis which it closely resembled. Macroscopically the brain is enlarged but histologically the tumour cell infiltration in the adventitial space of the vessels is clearly visible. With further growth the individual fields of infiltration can fuse and finally form small solid tumours visible with the naked eye. The leptomeninges are only secondarily infiltrated. Numerous mitoses with diffuse cell destruction and with conspicuous karyorrhexis is striking. The distinction between nuclear debris and mitosis is often difficult. Of our 4 cases, 3 were female and 1 was a male patient. The average age was higher, the youngest case being 40 years old and the oldest 64. The prognosis of our cases was bad and corresponded to that of glioblastoma. In differential diagnosis there were interesting relations with the reticuloendothelioses of the brain, e. g.: reticulosarcoma, but this can be discussed later.

3. *Sarcoma (arachnoidal) of the cerebellum* *: This group is the most poorly defined and is dependant on the description of *Foerster* and *Gagel* and a few cases in the literature (e. g. of *Marquardt* and *Neubuerger-Richter*). Infiltration of the leptomeninges is characteristic. From it the cells extend along the *Virchow-Robin* space on to the cerebellum. Histologically the tumour tissue can be recognized as islands of large pale cells lying close together with streaks of darkly staining lymphoid elements. There is a widespread reticulin network and especially around the foci where the leptomeninges are infiltrated with tumour. From the differential diagnostic point of view it must be emphasized that this tumour bears no relation to the sarcoma of the cerebellum described by *Zimmerman* and *Netsky* which appears to correspond exactly to the retothel sarcoma of *Rössle* and *Roulet.* Biologically we had in our 5 cases, 3 cases in men of middle age (40—50 years) and 2 women, including the youngest patient aged 16 years. As to the biological status we cannot say anything definite except that we are probably dealing with a malignant tumour.

4. *The Monstrocellular Sarcoma* **: This group was by far the largest in our series. It was described in detail by *Schmincke* in 1941 under the name ganglioglioneuroma. At that time the extra-

---

* *Schröder, M.,* Gibt es das umschriebene Arachnoidalsarkom des Kleinhirns von Foerster und Gagel? (Im Druck.)

** *Bingas, B.,* Das monstrozelluläre Sarkom. Arch. Psychiatr. (Im Druck.)

ordinary size of the cells (up to 340 μ and later up to 500 μ) was already emphasized. *Zülch* (1956) has tabulated the cases appearing in the literature up to 1935 (see p. 475).

This tumour has certain peculiarities which enable it to be distinguished from glioblastoma multiforme with the naked eye: the tumours have a rough appearance as if composed of asbestos fibres. They are mostly sharply demarcated like metastases, are firmer than the brain tissue often resembling meningiomas but are never "variegated". On the other hand they are often permeated by large cysts. The surrounding brain shows a marked brain swelling.

The tumour is histologically well characterized by the pleomorphism of the cells, which can range from small lymphoid or spindle elements up to monster cells of all sorts. These monsters can attain almost $^1/_2$ mm. and be visible with the naked eye. They contain large sheets of cytoplasm with 30—50 "nuclei" or cell inclusions. One can however see giant nuclear plaques almost without a definite nuclear body. The cells are often undergoing mitosis with the grossest abnormalities. Giant mitoses and amitotic division may also be seen. Sometimes the nuclei appear ganglioid which renders the original classification of the tumour by *Schmincke* comprehensible. The tumour has a tendency to liquefaction and mucoid degeneration and is relatively non-vascular. It is important to note that metastases occur in the extracranial organs e. g. heart and lungs, apart from direct infiltration of mesodermal tissues such as dura and bone.

In histological differential diagnosis, the formation of fibres between the cells and a network of fibre rings around the vessels is important. This permits us to consider the tumour as a genuine sarcoma of the vessels.

Biologically there is a preponderance of males to females in the ratio of 5 : 3. The sites of the tumour are distributed over the whole brain without any predilection and the age incidence is also very uncharacteristic extending from 5—80 years. The biological malignancy of the tumour is about that of the glioblastoma.

5. *Fibrosarcoma of the dura* *: There were certain points in common between the fibrosarcoma and meningiomas. They grow from the dura but are poorly demarcated from the brain. Brain swelling may be very marked. Histologically they are characterized by their spindle cell nature, the rich fibre formation and the presence of numerous mitoses. We had 30 cases of which 17 were in women and 13 in men. There was no site of predilection. The biological

---

* *Bingas, B.,* Das Fibrosarkom der Dura. (Im Druck.)

prognosis in these cases was bad. They have the same malignancy as the monstrocellular sarcomas. The line of distinction between these tumours and the malignant meningiomas is poorly defined.

6. *Reticulosarcomas* *: The small group of primary reticulosarcomas of the brain has also been discussed extensively since *Wilke* first described the peculiar and poorly defined demarcation between genuine primary sarcoma and reticulo-endotheliosis. In regard to our tumours we accept the definition of *Rössle* and *Roulet* for a reticulosarcoma: A reticular character with a close relationship of the tumour cells to the fine fibre net of silver fibrils, so that the cells are situated on the fibres like "pussy willow buds". The age incidence is that of middle life.

Biologically these tumours obviously have a better prognosis than that of most sarcomas.

In summary, we may say that out of the large and poorly defined field of brain sarcomas 6 groups may be indicated and defined thereby facilitating more complete discussion. A classification along these lines could be discussed when considering brain tumours as a whole.

* *Bingas, B.*, Retikulumzellsarkome des Gehirns. Zbl. Neurochir. (Im Druck.)

The Classification and Diagnosis of Intracranial Sarcomas

By

J. M. Brucher

With 4 Figures

In recent years we have been able to observe ten cases of primary intracranial sarcomas. Because of the rarity of these tumours and the varying opinions on their nature found in the literature, we have undertaken a more thorough study and we have endeavoured to classify them.

Zülch (1956) classified primary intracranial sarcomas as follows:

A. Cerebral sarcomas.
    1. Circumscribed sarcomas of the vessels ("Monstrocellular sarcomas").
    2. Diffuse vascular sarcomatosis ("Perivascular sarcomatosis. adventitial sarcoma or reticulosarcoma").
B. Meningeal sarcomas.
    1. Malignant meningiomas and fibrosarcomas of the dura mater.
    2. Circumscribed sarcomas of the cerebellar arachnoid.
    3. Diffuse leptomeningeal sarcomatosis.

In a more recent work, *Seitz* and *Kalm* (1958) have been able to confirm the existence of monstrocellular sarcomas, of adventitial sarcomas and of diffuse leptomeningeal sarcomatosis. This work deals with seven cases of monstrocellular sarcoma, two cases of perivascular sarcoma and one case of malignant meningioma. In addition, we have studied, in collaboration with Dr. *Vandeputte,* the neuropathological aspects of diffuse leptomeningeal sarcomatosis produced by the polyoma virus in the rat.

1. Monstrocellular sarcomas

The main clinical and macroscopical characteristics of the seven cases of circumscribed sarcomas of the vessels are listed in the table.

It is thus seen that patients of both sexes and all ages are subject to the disease in approximately the same manner. The course of the disease was always very rapid and the first symptoms appeared three to four weeks to four month prior to operation. On the average, post-operative survival was of several weeks duration but in one case attained sixteen months. The second patient survived only

Monstrocellular Sarcomas of the Brain

Name	Age Sex	Duration	Localisation	Appearance	General postmortem findings
vRa. H. 2074	♂ 9 yrs.	6 to 8 weeks	L. ant. temp.	Round, smooth, well demarcated, 5 cm. diam., greyish-pink, granular, hard. Cyst of C. S. F. gelatinous softening	Normal
He. B 5/60	♀ 23 yrs.	3 weeks + 11 months (oper × 2)	Deep left parietal	Smooth, well demarcated, 4 cm. diam., granular, firm. Easily enucleated. Oedema of neighbouring tissue.	—
Vers. H. 2098	♀ 24 yrs.	2 months + 16 months	Deep right frontal	Well defined, 5 cm. diam., Hard. Easily enucleated.	—
Bi. H. 2575	♂ 28 yrs.	1 month + 8 days		Well defined, 3 cm. diam., yellow, granular, firm	—
Hol. A 18/61	♀ 40 yrs.	1 month	Left putamen.	Well defined, round, 5 cm. diam., granular, hard, grey	Normal
Verv. B 122/60	♂ 52 yrs.	4 months + 6 weeks	Deep right post. temp.	Round, smooth, well defined, 5—6 cm. dia., yellow, hard. Oedema of neighbouring tissue	—
vHo. H. 2478	♀ 57 yrs.	3 months + 9 days	Right Rolandic	"Appearance of metastasis"	—
3 ♂ 4 ♀	9—57 yrs	4 + 16 months	Mostly right temp.	"Appearance of metastasis"	2 × norm.

eleven months although she underwent two surgical interventions, each of which was followed by radiotherapy.

In all cases the tumours were located deep in the cerebral hemisphere, most often in the frontal or temporal lobe. The macroscopic characteristics of these tumours are sufficiently constant for the diagnosis to be presumed by the neurosurgeon, at the moment of surgical intervention. Most often it is a round tumour, 3 to 6 cm. in diameter, whose well defined borders make total removal easy. The consistence of the tumour varies between firm and hard. It is often granular in its general appearance and of a greyish, yellowish or slightly pinkish colour. Small areas of gelatinous softening may be found in it. In one case the pressure of the ventricular temporal horn caused the formation of a cerebrospinal cyst in the neighbourhood of the tumour. In several instances, operation showed a marked oedema of the surrounding tissues.

This macroscopic appearance is often mistaken for that of a metastasis (Fig. 1). In two of the seven cases autopsy showed absence of any primary tumour outside the skull.

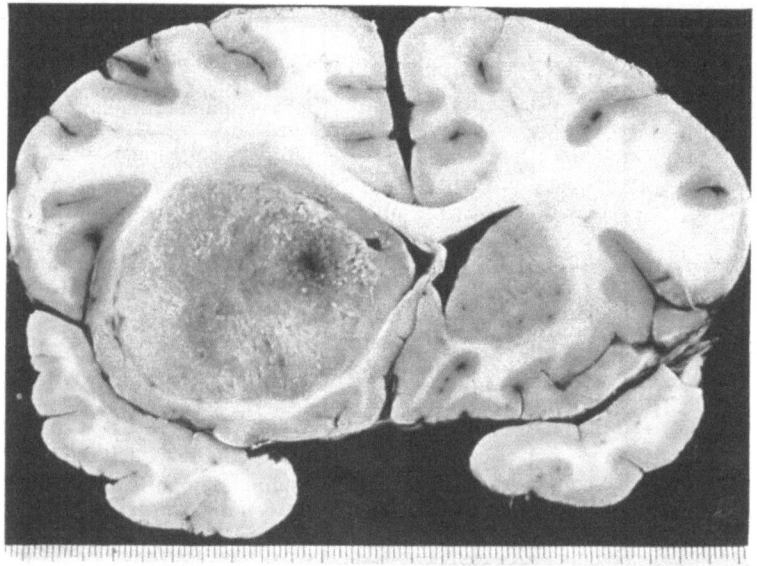

Fig. 1.

The microscopic picture is dominated by the presence of numerous giant cells with a pathognomic complex of special characteristics. These cells vary greatly in shape and sometimes possess amoeboid-like contours. They are so big that they may well be described as monstrous (Fig. 2). Actually their dimensions may attain 250 to 300 microns. The thick processes of the cell bodies often give them a similar appearance to those of large nerve cells. We seem to be dealing here with cells derived from fibroblasts since numerous elements of intermediate size seem to form a transition between typical fusiform fibroblasts and the giant cells.

The dense cytoplasm, takes eosin very well, has a spumous appearance and may contain vacuoles. Nuclei of varying size and sometimes very numerous, are dispersed haphazardly. Some contain rough chromatin blocks which stain very darkly. Others, on the other hand, are clear and vesicular. The nuclear membrane is very prominent. Most of these nuclei are characterized by the presence of one or two very large nucleoli of such a size as to make them resemble more closely nuclear inclusions. Some giant cells with filaments and containing a vesicular nucleus with a large nucleolus at the centre, look very much like hypertrophic nerve cells. Apart

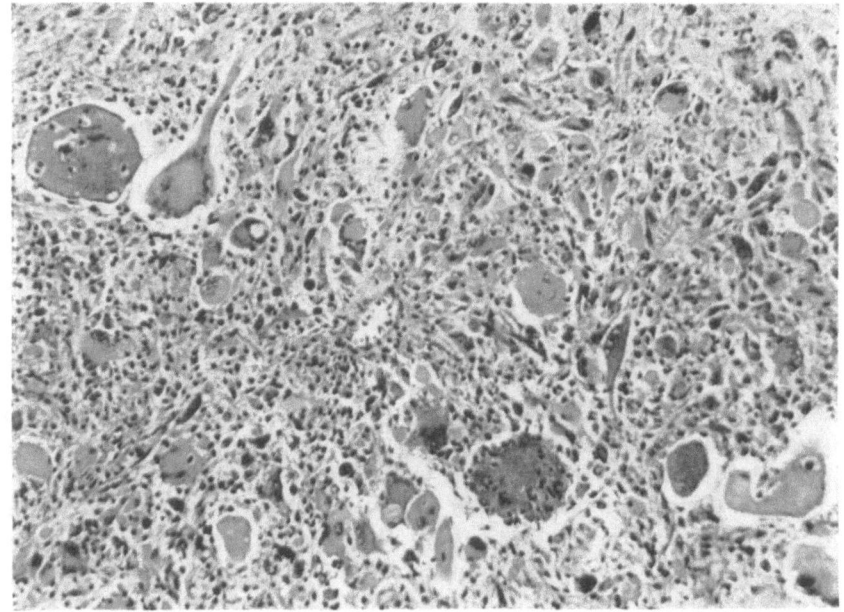

Fig. 2.

from their nuclei these giant cells often contain granular chromatic inclusions which seem to be phagocytosed leucocytes. Mitotic images were frequent and almost all abnormal.

The enormous size of these cells, the nerve cell-like appearance, the voluminous nucleoli, the phagocytic appearances and abnormal mitoses constitute a complex of characteristics which may be considered as pathognomonic for monstrocellular sarcomas. The giant cells which may be observed in certain gliomas, in particular in polymorphic oligodendrogliomas, present from time to time one or the other of these characteristics but these are never found together in the same case. The size of these giant glial cells is never greater than 150 microns. In addition, the crown-like arrangement of these nuclei as in the Langhans cells, and the filiform nuclear filaments so frequently found in certain gliomas and especially in polymorphic oligodendrogliomas, are almost never seen in sarcomas.

The giant cells are sometimes concentrated in areas while the fibroblastic cells organize themselves in other areas in the form of bundles with an obviously fibrous or fibro-sarcomatous aspect.

Among these polymorph cells, extending from the fibroblasts to the monstrous cells, via all the intermediary forms of giant fibroblasts, numerous cells of lymphoid type can be seen diseminated throughout the tumour, but mainly in a sheet-like arrangement around some of the vessels.

The vessels never show any endothelial proliferation except in the vicinity of necroses. This is a special characteristic which allows a fairly rapid distinction to be made from glioblastomas. On the other hand the vascular walls show a proliferation of adventitial cells which become progressively transformed into giant fibroblasts and monstrous cells. These cells arrange themselves tangentially or perpendicularly with respect to the vascular wall. Sometimes they are found along the lining of the vascular lumen, which seems to be devoid of all endothelium.

Silver impregnation techniques permit the demonstration of an intercellular network of reticulin fibrils. This proliferation increases around the vessels from which the reticulin radiates in all directions. In certain places, thicker reticulin fibers arrange themselves into bundles. It is important to note that certain segments, especially at the periphery of the tumour, even if they contain many monstrous cells, show no evidence of intercellular reticulin fibers. Possibly these areas are too young or insufficiently differentiated to be able to produce interstitial fibres. This observation is important because it prevents us from searching for absolute criteria for reticulin fibres in very small biopsies. Inversely, the presence of an interstitial reticulin network does not justify drawing an absolute conclusion as to the mesodermal origin of the tumour. It is actually well known that gliomas may invade the subarachnoidal spaces, proliferate abundantly there, and induce reactive production of interstitial collagen fibres. The confusion is particularly likely when the the tumour proliferates or grows within the depths of the sulcus giving the surgeon the impression that he is dealing with a deep tumour independent of the meninges. We were confronted with this difficulty when reviewing a series of polymorphic oligodendrogliomas in which the presence of giant cells, mitoses and

interstitial reticulin at first suggested the diagnosis of monstrocellular sarcoma. In these cases the cytological characteristics described above rather than the silver impregnation techniques permitted us to make the differential diagnosis of polymorphic oligodendroglioma. In addition, the slow evolution of these tumours
pleaded against their malignant nature. It remains a fact, however,
that the search for reticulin is an important argument in favour of
diagnosis, in particular in autopsy cases where histological examination may be made on fragments taken some distance away
from the meninges.

In the monstrocellular sarcoma several necrotic areas may exist
and these show a marked tendency to connective tissue scar-
formation in the middle of which may be seen, here and there, an
isolated giant cell. We have never seen any calcification.

The microscopic limits of the tumour are as clear as with the
naked eye. Several perivascular tumour cuffs penetrate for a short
distance within the very oedematous and spongy cerebral parenchyma. Large spaces around the dilated vessels and filled with
albuminous fluid may be seen in it. We have never observed isolated tumour cells within the healthy parenchyma as is seen around
gliomas. Sometimes the tumour reaches the brain surface and the
subarachnoidal spaces, where it proliferates in a circumscribed
manner.

These monstrocellular tumours thus show a series of macroscopic and microscopic characteristics which clearly distinguish
them. The great number of fusiform cells of the fibroblastic type
and of intermediary forms up to the monstrous cells, the presence
of interstitial reticulin in places which are definitely independent
of the arachnoidal membrane and finally the perivascular proliferation of the cells and of reticulin suggest that these tumours
are sarcomas, which develop from the vascular walls. These observations merely serve to confirm the earlier work of Professor.
Zülch to whom credit goes for distinguishing this type of tumour
in 1939 and 1940.

2. Diffuse Vascular Sarcomatosis

This form has been described more rarely. *Henschen* (1955)
estimated that only 35 to 40 cases have been published. It is difficult to get an exact idea of the number of cases published in the
literature for they are interpreted in very different fashions. *Lewy*
(1921) called them "diffuses Peritheliom" and thought already at
this time that they were sarcomas of the vascular walls. *Környey*

(1936) suggested the name "adventitial sarcomas" where as *Scheinker* (1936) preferred "diffuses perivasculäres Sarkom".

Many authors used the term "reticulum cell sarcoma" (*Yuile*, 1938), (*Kinney* and *Adams*, 1943), or "retothelsarkom" (*Gerhartz*, 1954) or even perithelioma (*Bailey*, 1929) and perithelial sarcoma (*Hsü*, 1940; *Hanbary* and *Dugger*, 1954). Metallic impregnation of tumour cells made *Benedek* and *Juba* (1941) as well as *Russell* and coll (1948), claim that microgliomas and microgliomatosis were involved.

Actually the tumour forms described under these names are not well defined. In many cases diffuse leptomeningeal sarcomatoses were involved, notably, with secondary invasion of the cerebral parenchyma. In addition, the confusion was increased when *Wilke* (1950), *Bertrand* and *Gruner* (1955) as well as *den Hartog* and coll. (1960) gathered under the same name ("reticulose" or "reticulo-endotheliosis") a series of encephalitic, granulomatous and neoplastic diseases. Even though the nomenclature is not of fundamental importance, it is essential to separate inflammatory from neoplastic diseases and to recognize the clinical and anatomical characteristics of the various forms of tumour.

That is the reason why I have sent you several histological specimens of the two cases which I have recently studied. In our view, one is an adventitial sarcoma (H 1885) in which the disease lasted only three months; the other, developed over 9 years and is a granulomatous reticulohistiocytic encephalitis (H 2039), such as *Cervós-Navarro* (1958) described.

One of the difficulties lies in the fact that the clinical picture and a superficial examination of the histological specimen may lead one to a diagnosis of encephalitis. Various authors and more recently still, *Draganescu* and coll. (1958) have underlined the pseudo-encephalitic aspect of the perivascular infiltrations.

In several cases in the literature, as in our case, the diffuse perivascular sarcomatosis is characterized, on the one hand, by one or more tumour areas, sometimes symmetrical and systematic in arrangement, and on the other by the perivascular extension of tumour cells throughout the white matter (Fig. 3), in the brain stem and ultimately in the cortex and the subarachnoidal spaces.

In these areas the tumour cells are often arranged in small groups as was already noted by *Mage* and *Scherer* (1937), *Wilke* (1950) and *Draganescu* and coll. (1958). These cell groups often have a capillary or fat-laden macrophage in the centre. They sometimes form synplasmas (syncytiums). The nuclei are round or highly polymorphic containing rough chromatin blocks and often

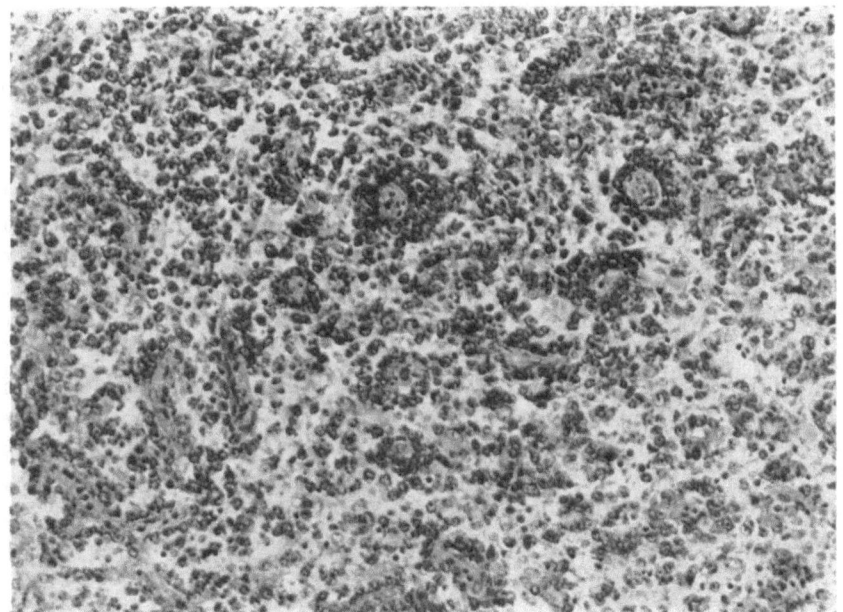

Fig. 3.

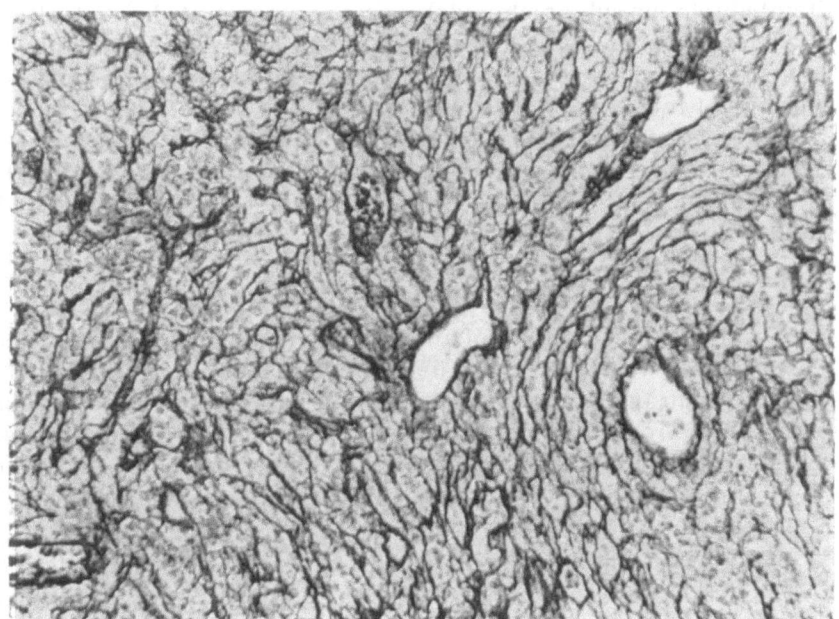

Fig. 4.

seem to be swollen. Many mitotic figures, amitoses, and nuclear remnants may be seen.

In several places the reticulin fibres form a delicate interstitial network (Fig. 4) and the reticulin proliferation is often limited to the neighbourhood of the vessels.

The infiltration of the white matter is very similar to that of perivenous encephalitis. At a greater magnification, the perivascular cuffs are seen to be formed chiefly by neoplastic cells showing the same blastomatous characteristics as in the main areas. Sometimes. lymphocytic and plasmocytic cells may be seen in it, and constitute secondary inflammatory reactions.

Recently we have been able to study, in biopsy, a new case of adventitial sarcoma. The patient was a woman of 44 when the disease began with headaches and mental disorders three and a half months prior to the operation. A soft tumour infiltrating the pre- and post-central cortex, and spreading deeply into the basal ganglia was discovered. The tumour was red and highly vascularized. Its border was poorly demarcated. Despite radiotherapy the patient died at home, four months after the operation. Examination of the biopsy showed a tumour of the white matter, which, in places, invaded the cortex and reached the pia mater. The tumour cells proliferated into the sub-arachnoidal spaces and penetrated even further into the cortex, along the vessels. As in the first case, the arrangement of the perivascular groups, the appearance of the neoplastic cells and of the reticulin network are typical of adventitial sarcomas.

These tumours proliferate from the vascular wall, as was already suggested by *Lewy* in 1921. For *Hanbery* and *Dugger* (1954), the neoplastic cells originate in multiplication of the undifferentiated mesenchymal cells of *Maximow*.

3. Malignant Meningiomas

We also studied a case of malignant meningioma. The patient was a man 58 years old whose first symptoms began one and a half years prior to the operation. The surgeon was able to remove a big parasagittal frontal tumour adherent to the dura mater and to the superior longitudinal sinus. It penetrated to a great depth within the brain but remained well demarcated and encapsulated as would a meningioma.

The microscopical examination revealed the classical structure of the meningioma but there were areas characterized by numerous multinucleated cells, by large hyperchromatic nuclei and by normal and abnormal mitosis.

4. Diffuse Leptomeningeal Sarcomatosis

Finally, I would like to show you, rapidly, the neuropathological aspects of diffuse leptomeningeal sarcomatosis produced experimentally by means of the polyoma virus in the rat. This result was obtained in 1960 by *Rabson* and *Kirschtein* by the intracerebral inoculation of this virus into the hamster. Recently, my colleague, Dr. *M. C. Vandeputte*, was able to produce the same tumour in the rat using either intra-venous or subcutaneous as well as intracerebral inoculations.

A diffuse neoplastic process of the pia-mater is involved, predominant in the lower part of the brain and invading the cerebral parenchyma either along the vessels or in a diffuse manner. The tumour cells seem to originate in the proliferation of the pia mater and are of a clearly fibroblastic nature. There is abundant reticulin formation and there are numerous mitotic images.

This diffuse tumour may cause haemorrhagic infiltrations, haemorrhages, and even hydrocephalus.

This neoplastic process is entirely comparable to the diffuse leptomeningeal sarcomatosis which is rarely seen in man. The viral etiology of this experimental tumour opens new perspectives for the understanding and study of human sarcomas.

References

Bailey, P., Intracranial sarcomatous tumors of leptomeningeal origin. Arch. Surg. *18* (1929), 1359—1402. — *Benedek, L.*, and *A. Juba*, Über das Mikrogliom. Dtsch. Zschr. Nervenhk. *152* (1941), 159—169. — *Bertrand, I.*, and *J. Gruner*, Sur quelques types de granulomes et réticuloses de l'encéphale. Proceedings of the second International Congress of Neuropathology, London. Excerpta, Part II. Session X (1955), 362—364. — *Brucher, J. M*, and *E. Matthys*, A propos d'une observation d'encéphalite granulomateuse réticulo-histocytaire. Acta neurol. psychiatr. Belg. *60* (1960), 943—954. — *Cervós-Navarro, J.*, Encephalitis granulomatosa reticulohistiocitaria. Trab. Inst. Cajal Sec. fisiol., Madrid, *49* (1958), 123. — *Cervós-Navarro, J.*, *G. Hübner*, *G. Puchstein* and *A. Stammler*, Die Pathomorphologie der reticulo-histiocytären granulomatösen Encephalitis. Frankf. Zschr. Path. *70* (1960), 458—477. — *Draganescu, St.*, *S. Voinescu*, *Ar. Petrescu* and *N. Draganescu*, Proces neoformativ difuz cu aspecte encefalitice. Studii si cercetari de Neurologie *3*, 4 (1958), 375—385. — *Gehuchten (Van) P.*, and *J. M. Brucher*, Sarcome cérébral à localisations multiples et à extension périvasculaire diffuse, pouvant donner l'aspect d'une encéphalite. Rev. neurol., Paris, *102* (1960). 671—681. — *Gerhartz, H.*, Retothelsarcom des Zentralnervensystems. Virchows Arch. path. Anat. *319* (1951), 339—346. — *Hanbery, J. W.*, and *G. S. Dugger*, Perithelial sarcoma of the brain. Arch. Neurol. Psychiatr., London, *71* (1954). 732—761. — *Hartog (Den) J. C.*, *G. C. Guazzi* and *A. Nunes Vicente*, Réticulo endothéliose cérébrale primitive (dite encéphalite granulomateuse) et granulome infundibulo-tubérien. Rev. neurol., Paris, *102* (1960), 20—43. — *Henschen, F.*, Tumoren des Zentralnervensystems und seiner Hüllen. Hd. d. spez. pathol. Anat. u. Histol., Berlin. *13*. 3 (1955), 643—647. — *Hsü. Y. K.*, Primary intracranial sarcomas. Arch. Neurol. Psychiatr., London, *43* (1940), 901—924. — *Kinney, T. D.*, and *R. D. Adams*, Reticulum-cell sarcoma of the brain. Arch. Neurol. Psychiatr., London, *50* (1943), 552—564. — *Környey, S.*, Eine sich entlang den Gefäßwandungen ausbreitende Hirngeschwulst (adventitielles Sarkom). Zschr. Neurol., Berlin, *149* (1933), 50—67. — *Lewy, F. H.*, Die Lymphräume des Gehirns, ihr Bau und ihre Geschwülste. Virchows Arch. path. Anat. *232* (1921), 400—432. — *Mage, J.*, and *H. J. Scherer*, Tumeur cérébrale parvicellulaire se propageant dans l'espace de Virchow-Robin. J. belge neurol. psychiatr. *37* (1937), 731—746. — *Rabson, A.*, and *R. Kirschstein*, Intracranial sarcomas produced by polyoma virus in syrian hamsters. Amer. Med. Ass. Arch. Path. *69* (1960), 663—671. — *Russell, D. S., A. H. E. Marshall* and *F. B. Smith*, Microgliomatosis: a form of reticulosis affecting the brain. Brain, London, *71* (1948), 1—15. — *Scheinker, I.*, Über eine seltene zerebrale Tumorart (Diffuses perivasculäres Sarkom), mit besonderer Lokalisation im Stirnhirn. Jb. Psychiatr. Neurol. *53* (1936), 155—163. — *Seitz, D.*, and *H. Kalm*, Zur Diagnose der primären Hirnsarkome. Dtsch. Zschr. Nervenhk. *177* (1958), 597—617. — *Vandeputte, M. C.*, Lésions cérébrales chez le rat, induites par le virus polyome. Rev. belge path. *28* (1961), 178—183. — *Vandeputte, M. C.*, and *J. M. Brucher*, Sarcomatose méningée expérimentale provoquée chez le raton par le virus polyome. Acta neuropath. *1* (1962), 397 to 405. — *Wilke, G.*, Über primäre Reticuloendotheliosen des Gehirns. Dtsch. Zschr. Nervenhk. *164* (1950), 332—380. — *Yuile, C. L.*, Case of primary reticulum-cell sarcoma of the brain: relation of microglia cells to histiocytes. Arch. Path. Chicago, *26* (1938), 1036—1044. — *Zülch, K. J.*, Pathologische Anatomie der raumbeengenden intrakraniellen Prozesse. Hdb. d. Neurochir. Bd. III, Springer-Verlag, Berlin, 1956. 800 pages.

Microgliomatosis

By

L. J. Rubinstein

With 12 Figures

In 1948, *Dorothy Russell, Marshall* and *Smith* [10] reported under the title of "Microgliomatosis, a form of reticulosis affecting the brain", seven cases with a focal tumor-like proliferation of cells of predominantly microglial type. In four cases, the process was confined to the brain. In three, similar proliferations were present in other organs, including the cervical glands, spleen, kidney, parotid, bone-marrow and lungs. In the brain, the macroscopically visible infiltrates were either single or multiple, involving the cerebrum, basal ganglia, brain stem or cerebellum. The microscopic characteristics of the cerebral lesions consisted in: 1. The presence of extensive microscopic foci of cellular proliferation beyond the macroscopically defined borders of the main tumor masses. 2. An extensive infiltration, by tumor cells, of the Virchow-Robin spaces, with well-marked lymphocytic cuffings further afield, mimicking an encephalitis. 3. The cytological similarity of many of these cells to adult microglia of the brain or to histiocytes elsewhere in the body, with the presence of more primitive elements of the reticulo-endothelial system, regarded as reticulum cells. 4. A positive impregnation of the more differentiated cell elements by silver techniques specific for the mature macrophage system (Weil-Davenport, or Penfield's modification of Hortega's silver carbonate method for microglia), with a more feeble impregnation of the less differentiated elements.

These lesions were therefore, on the basis of silver techniques, interpreted as being largely composed of neoplastic cells with the morphological characteristics of microglia and their precursors, hence the term microglioma or microgliomatosis. Their relation to the more primitive reticulum-cell sarcoma was envisaged, and the view favored that the more primitive cell elements in these tumors arose from the de-differentiation of the more mature forms. However. the alternative possibility cannot be disregarded, namely that these tumors may histogenetically arise from more primitive elements, possibly undifferentiated periadventitial reticulum cells, and that the more mature microglial forms may represent their differentiated descendants. It is, however, difficult to see how this problem can be resolved with the present techniques.

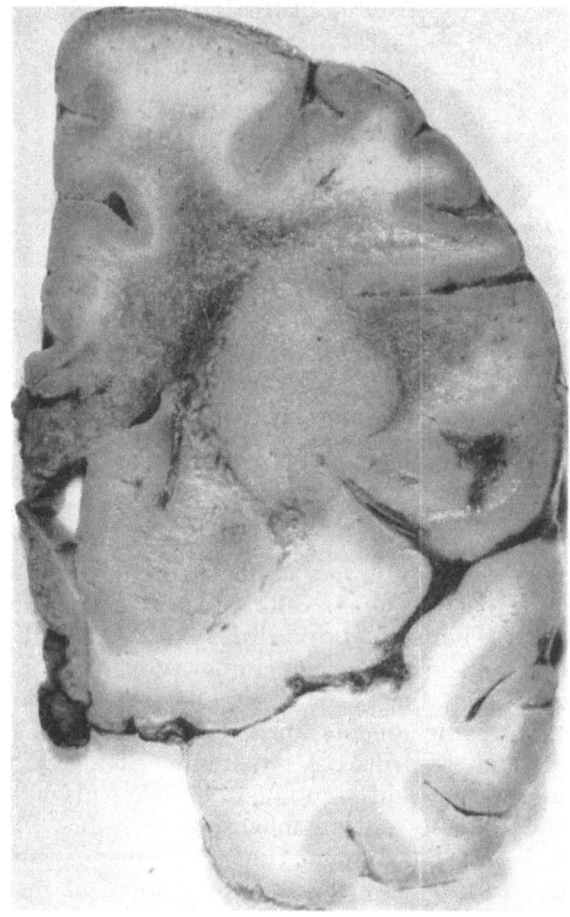

Fig. 1. Microgliomatosis. Case 1. Homogenous tumor mass in right frontal centrum ovale, with darker softer band of infiltration in remainder of white matter and corpus callosum.

A survey of the literature antecedent to *Russell's* paper indicated that similar cases had been described before, in particular by *Bailey*[1], *Benedek* and *Juba*[2], *Yuile*[13], and *Kinney* and *Adams*[6] In these examples, silver impregnation for microglia had been positive in many areas of the tumor, a finding which had led *Benedek* and *Yuile* to accept their essentially microglial nature. On the other hand, this interpretation, though considered by them, was rejected by *Bailey* and by *Kinney* and *Adams,* their cases being classified as perithelial sarcoma by the former and reticulum-cell sarcoma by the latter. *Russell* and coll. also suggested that many of the cases previously reported as "peritheliomas", "perithelial sarcomas" and "alveolar sarcomas" might well fall into the category of micro-

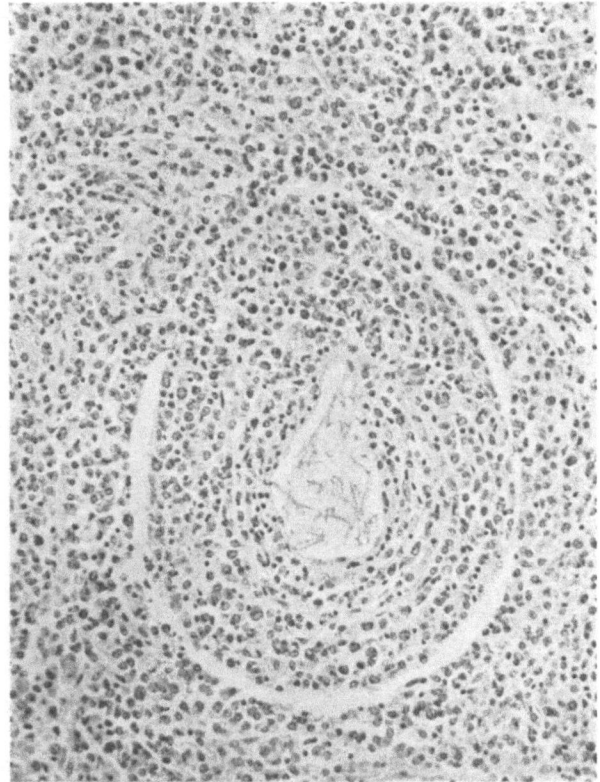

Fig. 2. Case 1. Highly cellular infiltrate of main tumor mass, distending the Viichow-Robin space. H. and E. 200 ×.

gliomas, but in the absence of specific silver impregnations it was impossible to be sure of this. The same uncertainty exists in the case of examples reported more recently in the literature as "primary reticulum cell sarcoma[7]". Thus, the interesting case presented, and reported elsewhere, by Dr. *Brucher*[11] as a cerebral sarcoma with diffuse perivascular extensions seems to me indistinguishable

from some of our own examples of diffuse microgliomatosis. In
the absence of silver impregnations, however, this question cannot,
I believe, be resolved with complete assurance. Where, however,
these have been performed, support for this interpretation has been
gained, as for instance in the cases reported by *Fisher* and coll.[5]
in 1959, and classified by these workers as "reticulum-cell sarcomas
(microgliomas)". Examination of our own subsequent tumor material in London by silver methods has not only confirmed this
interpretation, but also indicated that there may be an appreciable

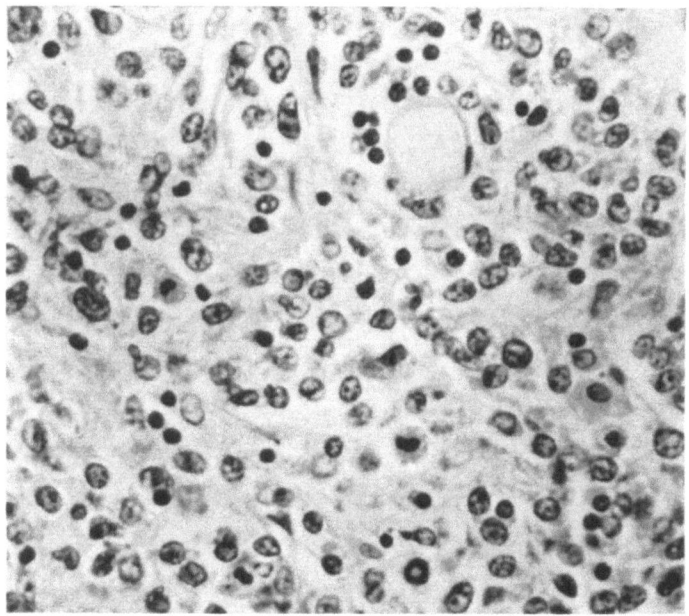

Fig. 3. Case 1. Cellular detail of tumor infiltrate. H. and E. 400 ×.

measure of variation within this group in general, in respect to the
proportion of silver-impregnated tumor cells and particularly in
regard to their capacity to stimulate a connective-tissue stroma.
Three fairly recent examples examined by us have been circulated
on the occasion of this Symposium, and the following illustrations,
selected from two of them, recapitulate their principal features.

Figs. 1 to 7 demonstrate the appearances in the case of a woman
of 57, with a three weeks' history of headaches, drowsiness and
progressive mental changes. At necropsy (courtesy of Prof. *P. M.
Daniel*, London), the brain revealed a diffuse infiltration of both
frontal centra ovalia by firm gray granular tissue, bordered by a

widespread zone of softer, more crumbly tissue which spread into the remainder of the frontal white matter and crossed over the corpus callosum (Fig. 1). Microscopically, the main mass consisted in a dense aggregate of tumor cells which, as indicated in Fig. 2, frequently filled the greatly dilated Virchow-Robin spaces. Under higher power (Fig. 3), the cells displayed a thin, very ill-defined rim of cytoplasm, with single round or oval nuclei, occasionally lobed or indented, surrounded by a well defined nuclear membrane and presenting a pale nucleoplasm and a moderate chromatin mesh-

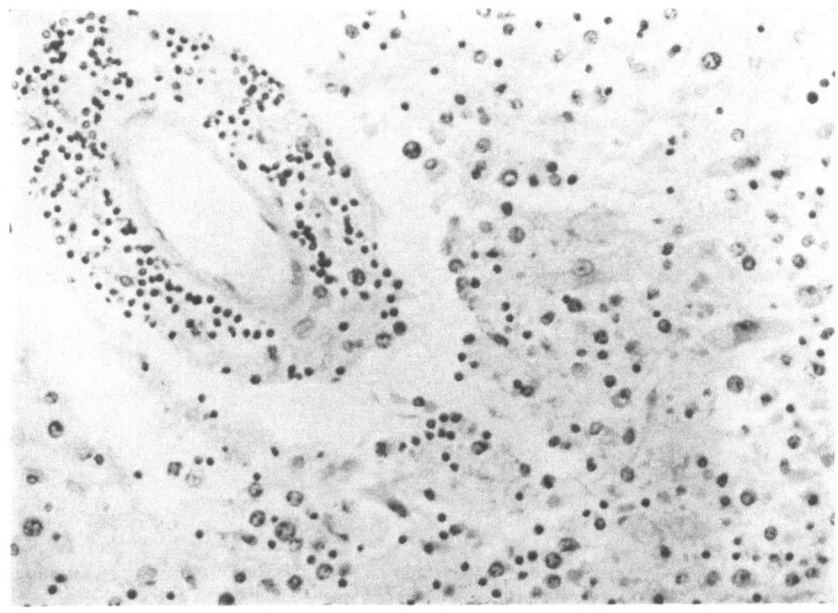

Fig. 4. Case 1. Less densely cellular area. More pleomorphic cell-infiltrate, adjacent to a blood vessel showing largely lymphocytic perivascular cuffing. Two reactive astrocytes are present near the right margin of the field. H. and E. 300 ×.

work with, sometimes, a single nucleolus. Mitoses were numerous. In the softer peripheral zone noted macroscopically, the cellular density was less intense and the cytology more pleomorphic, consisting, in addition to the above-mentioned cells, in a mixture of inflammatory cells of lymphocytic and plasmocytic type. The perivascular distribution of the tumor cells was, however, well maintained, though, in places, the perivascular cuffs were largely lympho-cytic (Fig. 4). A marked astrocytic gliosis was present in this area. In addition, the overlying cortical leptomeninges were extensively infiltrated by cells which were morphologically similar to those already described, mixed with a small number of lymphocytes and plasma cells. The superficial cortical layer beneath the meningeal infiltration showed also a focal accumulation of similar cells. The reticulin preparations revealed a slight to moderate diffuse increase of reticulin, with a perivascular distribution which we have now come to regard as characteristic of microgliomatosis. As depicted in Fig. 5, this consists in a concentric increase of the perivascular reticulin, with a lacy pattern of more rarefied broken fibers, which forms a delicate network limited externally by the well-defined outer pial membrane of the infiltrated and distended Virchow-Robin

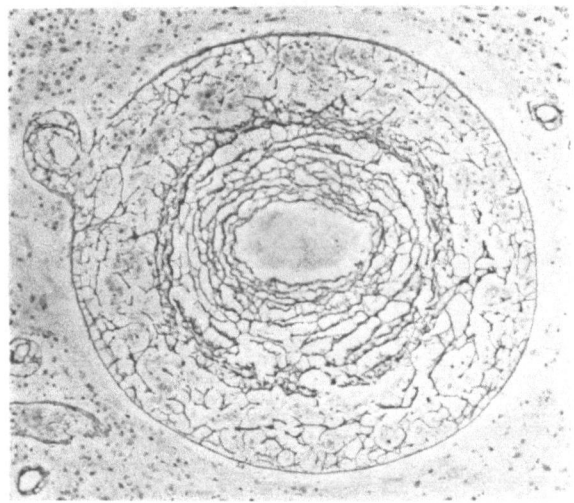

Fig. 5. Case 1. Characteristic pattern of increased perivascular reticulin fibers in greatly dilated Virchow-Robin space. Gomori's reticulin method 80 ×.

space. Silver preparations for microglia demonstrated an intense metalophilia of a large proportion of the tumor cells (Fig. 6), whose cytoplasmic outline could then be clearly visualized, presenting the typical appearance of activated microglia, often with short cytoplasmic processes (Fig. 7). A proportion of tumor cells in both Virchow-Robin spaces and leptomeninges were similarly impregnated by silver.

Figs. 8 to 12 illustrate the features of the case in a man of 57, with a twelve months' history of headaches and the onset, six weeks before death, of progressive mental deterioration and left lower limb paresis. At necropsy (courtesy of Dr. *D. R. Oppenheimer*, Oxford), a fairly well defined firm gray granular tumor was found to occupy the right orbital cortex and white matter, locally infiltrating

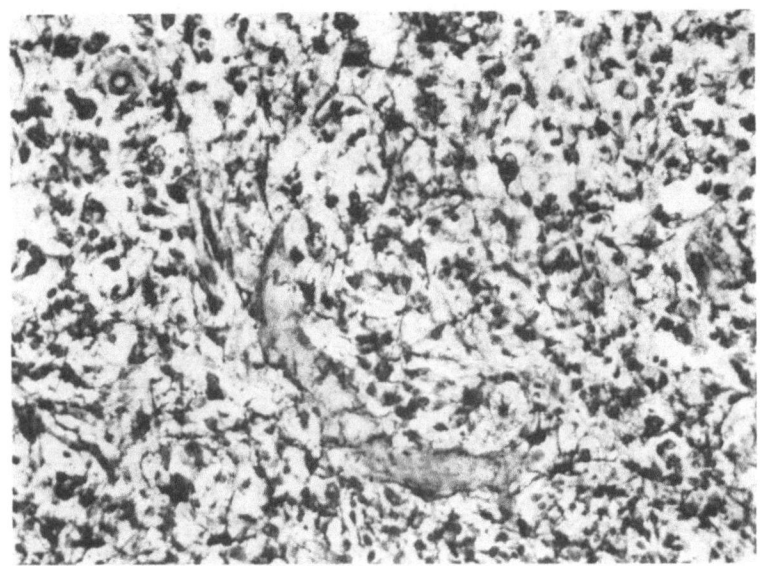

Fig. 6. Case 1. Positive silver impregnation of many tumor cells. Penfield's modification of Hortega's silver carbonate method for microglia. 200 ×.

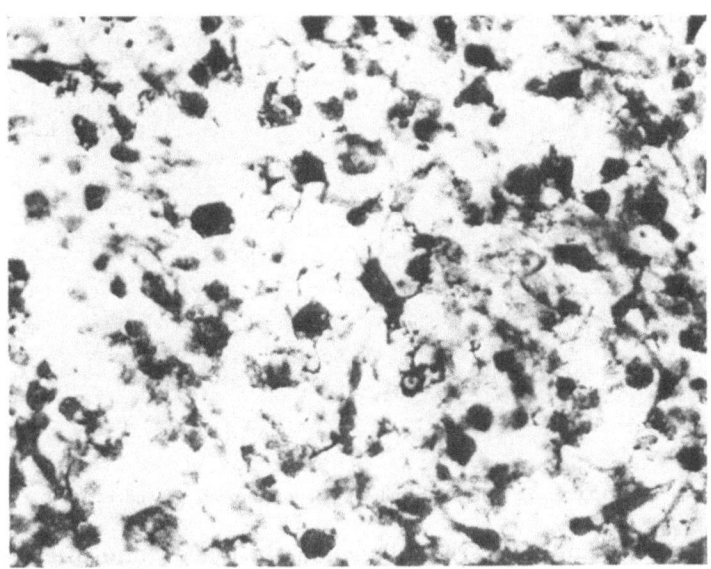

Fig. 7. Case 1. Morphological details of silver-impregnated cells, microglial in character. Penfield's modification of Hortega's silver carbonate for microglia. 400 ×.

the leptomeninges (Fig. 8). As shown in Fig. 9, the cytology of the tumor was essentially similar to that of the previous case. This tumor showed, however, an unusually abundant and dense fibrous

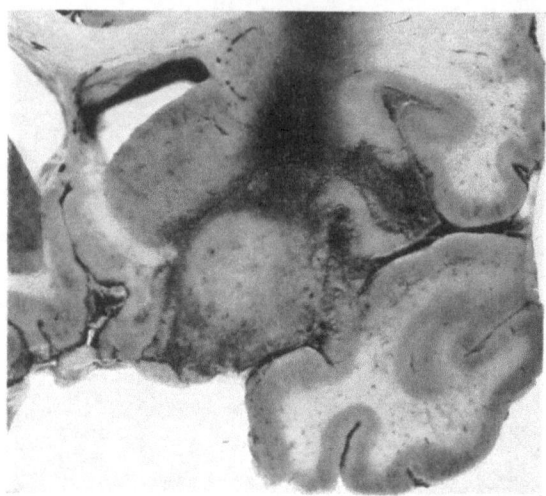

Fig. 8. Microgliomatosis. Case 2. Homogenous gray tumor replacing the orbital cortex and white matter, and infiltrating the underlying leptomeninges. The hemorrhages are the result of recent surgical trauma.

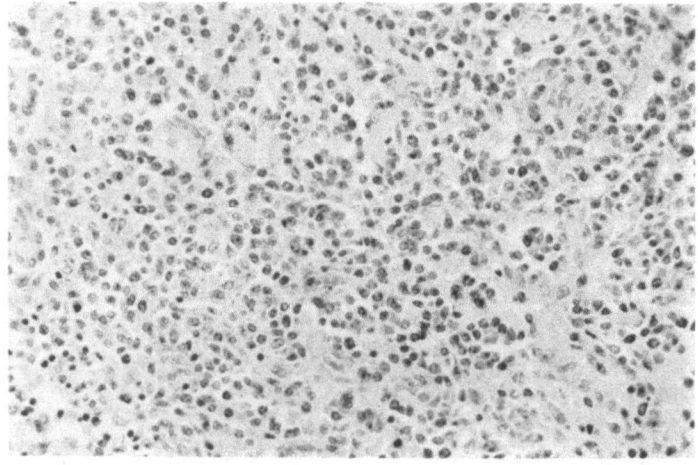

Fig. 9. Case 2. Cellular morphology of tumor mass. H. and E. 200 ×.

connective-tissue network, collagenous in places, and often separating tumor cells into islands of various sizes (Fig. 10); elsewhere, the classical perivascular increase of reticulin depicted in Fig. 5 was also observed. Silver impregnations for microglia again revealed an intense metalophilia of many of the tumor cells (Fig. 11), with, under the higher power, the characteristic morphological appearances of activated microglia (Fig. 12).

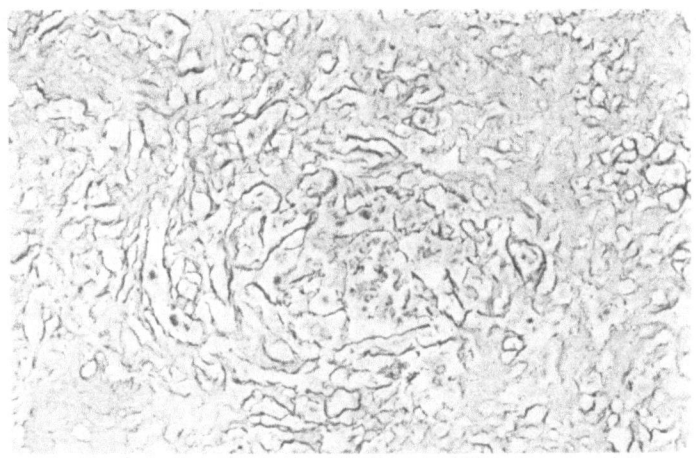

Fig. 10. Case 2. Considerable increase of fibrous connective tissue (reticulin and collagen) separating small pale islands of tumor cells. Gomori's reticulin method 170 ×.

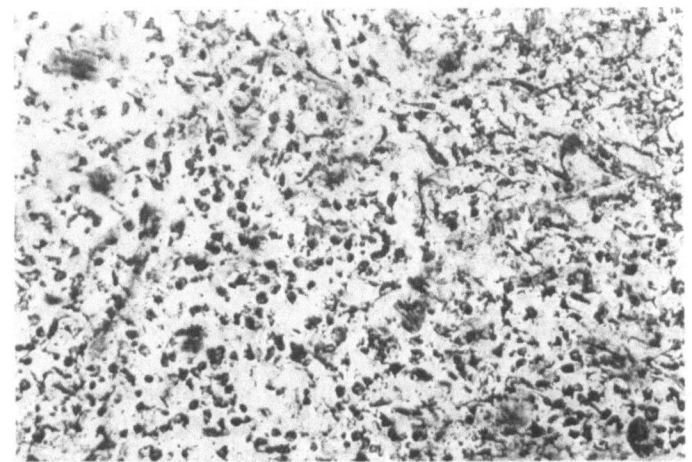

Fig. 11. Case 2. Positive silver impregnation of many tumor cells. Penfield's modification of Hortega's silver carbonate methode for microglia. 200 ×

I would now like to touch briefly upon the relation of these tumors to the lymphomas in general and to the cases described by *Wilke*[12], *Cervós-Navarro*[4] and *Brucher*[3] as "reticulo-histocytic

encephalilis". The examples which we have labelled "microgliomas"
are unquestionably neoplastic in nature. However, their frequent
association with similar proliferations in other parts of the body,
especially in organs of the reticulo-endothelial system, and the fact
that they implicate, in the brain, the elements regarded as a part
of the same system, have prompted us to regard them essentially as
falling among the neoplastic reticuloses, in the sense used by *Robb-
Smith* [9] and *Marshall* [8]. Some authorities would therefore simply
include these tumors among the general group of malignant

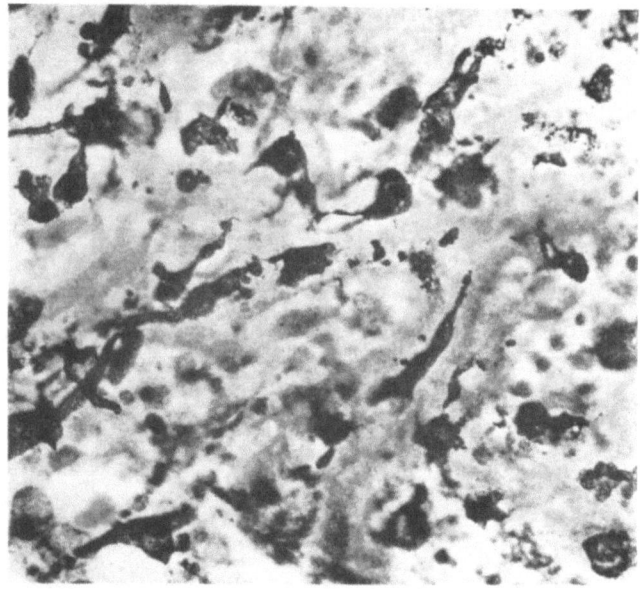

Fig. 12. Case 2. Morphology of tumor cells typical of activiated microglia in silver impregnation. Penfield's modification of Hortega's silver carbonate method for microglia. 400 ×.

lymphomas, a view with which our own classification is essentially
in agreement.

Dr. *Brucher* has, on the other hand, forcibly raised the question
of the relationship of the neoplasias affecting the reticulo-endothelial system in the brain, to those controversial entities of which
his example of "reticulo-histiocytic encephalitis" seems to be one [3].
He has favored a clear separation, in this general group, of those
cases which exhibit an essentially neoplastic picture from those
where the inflammatory cellular elements predominate. Such a
separation is, however, by no means clear-cut, since the existence
of transitional forms seems well authenticated [12]. From the illus-

trations of his case report [3] and from the slides he has circulated, I would much more favor the view that his is another example of a diffuse neoplastic reticulosis affecting the brain, and not a granulomatous inflammatory process. In a number of areas, there is a marked similarity to some of the examples which we have interpreted as microgliomatosis, and the resemblance is strengthened by the characteristic reticulin pattern presented in his preparations.

I would therefore suggest that the debate, which, like *Fisher* [5], I would regard as largely semantic, could perhaps be resolved if we consider these proliferative disorders of the reticulo-endothelial system in the brain within the context of the reticuloses and lymphomatous proliferations as they obtain in general pathology. For here too, we come across similar inherent problems of classification; these have recently been exhaustively reviewed by *Marshall* [8] (pp. 63 to 80) in his outline of the cytology and pathology of the reticular tissue. Thus he has emphasized (p. 65) that "the distinction between neoplasia or inflammatory hyperplasia in the reticular tissues is of the utmost difficulty on histological grounds, as in both processes the reacting cells are derived from the same tissue". Viewed in this light, the problem may then be removed from the sterile arena of semantic disputation and transferred to a more profitable domain, in which the essential nature of the lesions themselves, as manifested in the general group of the reticuloses, may be explored on the basis of their etiology.

References

1. *Bailey, P.,* Intracranial Sarcomas of Leptomeningeal Origin. Arch. Surg., Chicago, *18* (1929), 1357. — 2. *Benedek, L.,* and *A. Juba,* Über das Mikrogliom. Dtsch. Zschr. Nervenhk. *152* (1941), 159. — 3. *Brucher, J. M.,* and *E. Matthys.* A propos d'une observation d'encéphalite granulomateuse réticulo-histiocytaire. Acta neurol. psychiatr. Belg. *60* (1960), 943. — 4. *Cervós-Navarro, J.,* Encephalitis granulomatosa reticulohistiocitaria. Trab. Inst. Cajal Sec. fisiol., Madrid, *49* (1958). — 5. *Fisher, E. R., E. R. Davis* and *L. J. Lemmer,* Reticulum-Cell Sarcoma of the Brain (Microglioma). Arch. Neurol. Psychiatr., Chicago, *81* (1959), 591. — 6. *Kinney, T. D.,* and *R. D. Adams,* Reticulum Cell Sarcoma of the Brain. Arch. Neurol. Psychiatr., Chicago, *50* (1943), 552. — 7. *Losli, E. J.,* Primary Intracerebral Pleomorphic Reticulum-Cell Sarcoma. Arch. Path., Chicago, *64* (1956), 322. — 8. *Marshall, A. H. E.,* An Outline of the Cytology and Pathology of the Reticular Tissue. Oliver and Boyd, Edinburgh and London, 1956. — 9. *Robb-Smith, A. H. T.,* In: Recent Advances in Clinical Pathology. Ist Edition. Churchill, London, 1947. — 10. *Russell, D. S., A. H. E. Marshall* and *F. B. Smith,* Microgliomatosis. A Form of Reticulosis affecting the Brain. Brain. London, *71* (1948), 1. — *Van Gehuchten, P.,* and *J. M. Brucher,* Sarcome cérébral à localisations multiples et à extension périvasculaire diffuse pouvant donner l'aspect d'une encéphalite. Rev. neurol., Paris, *102* (1960), 671. — 12. *Wilke, G.,* Über primäre Reticuloendotheliosen des Gehirns. Dtsch. Zschr.

Nervenhk. *164* (1950), 332. — 13. *Yuile, C. L.*, Case of Primary Reticulum Cell Sarcoma of the Brain: Relation of Microglia Cells to Histiocytes. Arch. Path , Chicago, *26* (1938), 1036.

Discussion

Dr. Zülch: To open the discussion, Dr. Netsky, may I ask you to comment on Dr. Zimmermann's and your cerebellar sarcoma, because I very boldly put it into the reticular sarcomas in keeping with your atlas.

Dr. Netsky: It is entirely possible that what has been described as a cerebellar sarcoma is indeed a reticulum cell sarcoma. I judge by this you mean a variety of malignant lymphoma.

Dr. Zülch: Yes.

Dr. Netsky: Then I would concede that this may be so but once again I have not proved it and until I have better evidence than a histologic slide, I say really I don't know. The reason we chose the name cerebellar sarcoma — recognizing that this is not a good name — was to keep it indiscriminate as regards its actual nature. We might have called it a fibrous sarcoma if we thought it was this, or a reticulum cell sarcoma. I am inclined to think it more likely to be a reticulum cell sarcoma, but I can't be sure, and I don't believe anyone can.

Dr. Zülch: Thank you, Dr. Netsky. We just wanted for practical purposes to make a distinction between your type of cerebellar sarcoma and Foerster and Gagel's type of cerebellar arachnoidal sarcoma which has been reported in the literature by several contributors. I said we have 5 cases of this type of sarcoma, but I am not sure that they actually correspond to Gagel's tumour which I have never seen myself though I spent some time with Gagel and I wonder if this is a well defined entity at all. But the form of tumour which corresponds most closely to Gagel's description is the one we showed you. Perhaps Dr. Rubinstein has some opinion about it or has anyone else seen such a tumour?

Dr. Rubinstein: Yes, I have, but I was not going to discuss them because there is so much else to discuss. This is an extremely complicated problem, and I think I can superimpose these cases of Gagel upon those I have seen myself, but I don't think it would take us very far just now.

Dr. Zülch: I think we can dismiss then Gagel's arachnoidal sarcoma, perhaps we can agree about the type of diffuse meningeal sarcomatosis.

Dr. Rubinstein: I am sorry, Dr. Zülch, I think we are somewhat confused because I must say that...

Dr. Zülch: I just wanted for practical purposes to dismiss those, that we can't solve today. With others we have a certain amount of agreement and to have time for those types which we want really ...

Dr. Rubinstein: Yes, we could do so, but the point is that I am not quite sure from the preparations shown to us as to what I would call them if I saw them. I must confess that none of the pictures I have seen has the diagnosis I would give it, at least not at first glance. I think there are some diffuse sarcomas of the meninges such as those which Black and Kernohan have described. I have seen these too, but I did not think that the first three slides resembled those. In fact was there a difference between your first and second group as shown here with the perivascular arrangement? I could not see any.

Dr. Zülch: The first starts in the meninges and grows into the brain secondarily. The other one is starting in the depth of the brain and grows from there to the outside. It may infiltrate the meninges as the first may infiltrate the brain. It is the starting point, the primary location, which makes the difference.

Dr. Rubinstein: I recognize fibrosarcomas of the dura. The dura can form a sarcoma with fibre-producing cells which look highly malignant and which are easily recognisable by anyone, although again I was a bit embarrassed because the picture of the case you showed is not the typical picture of a fibrosarcoma.

Dr. Zülch: Then let us have some suggestions as to which groups we want to discuss this afternoon?

Dr. Rubinstein: Well, should we group, should we in fact make any formal division into groups?

Dr. Zülch: I agree this is a problem but we must have time to speak about granular histiocytic encephalitis and from there return to the adventitial sarcoma or the whole complex of similar tumours, because many of you are prepared to discuss these.

Dr. Rubinstein: Yes, perhaps this ought to be discussed.

Dr. Zülch: And secondly if anybody wishes to we can discuss the monstrocellular sarcomas. What do you think?

Dr. Woolf: I certainly think we should, because you got such a very much larger collection of them than say Rubinstein has.

Dr. Zülch: To start the discussion I hope everybody agrees that we begin with Dr. Bruchers paper.

Dr. Sayre: Excellent.

Dr. Zülch: I think it is really a paper which gives us a wealth of observations for discussion, which is open now. Dr. Rubinstein or Dr. Sayre, would you like to comment on this?

Dr. Sayre: I don't consider myself a specialist in sarcomas of the brain but my impression, however is that there are two types of tumours. The one that Dr. Brucher sent around was a reticulum cell sarcoma. My feeling was that it was the microgliomatous type of reticulum cell sarcoma; my feeling about the other was that I could not make it into a sarcoma as it seemed more to resemble an inflammatory disease. And I think this fits well with the clinical story.

Dr. Zülch: Thank you, Dr. Sayre. Dr. Netsky, you want to give your discussion?

Dr. Netsky: I agree with Dr. Rubinstein that the sarcomas like the gliomas are difficult, but that the sarcomas are even more difficult. It would be my natural inclination as one can understand from the proceedings of the last few days to agree with his concept, to accept as a working concept the diffuse reticular endothelioses which may have various manifestations. I would like to comment on this problem of classification, because I am just as guilty of misusing the word classification. On this ground I think that a proper classification or an ideal classification would be one that is first of all a rational one, that is, based on important and fundamental principles. If I were asked to classify the animals studied by Dr. Luginbühl and I listed dogs, cats, monkeys, horses, pigs and so on, he would say this is not a classification, it is merely a list. If I look at the "classification" Dr. Hamperl gave us I find I am expected to go from cells to tissues to organs; there is no rational basis. I hear Dr. Zülch say that one of the sarcomas in his "classification" is different from the other, that one begins in the meninges and extends to the cortex, the other begins in the cortex and extends to the meninges. Is this important? If I had a streptococcus abscess in my brain it might go from my scalp inward or from the brain outward, but still, knowing the organism, I say this is a streptococcal abscess and the mode of extension would not make any basic difference. Similarly when the diphtheritic organism causes a polyneuritis and demyelination, or a pharyngitis or meningitis the same organism is the cause. The important thing is that we know the aetiological agent in some cases. Classification should be rational, and I find no reason in what has been offered. I think this is largely due to our lack of information. We need much more information than we have. And then to split off the monstrocellular sarcoma! Is that truly different from other sarcomas? Is the presence of large cells an important difference or is it merely a descriptive detail. I would also ask if classification is to be rational that it be consistent. Let us not shift from one basis to another, such as age or sex or size of cell. It is furthermore important to have useful classifications. When we get a list like this, it is not useful for me because I can't remember these things, I try, but find it extremely difficult. If some fundamental principle could be found to unite the tumours then we would have a good classification. We would have it for sarcomas and gliomas, but as things stand now, we have no such thing. We do have a long list of different tumours. We can add many more and probably will, before we get some unifying principle. I hope that in succeeding meetings we will find unifying principles and not descriptions however elegant. I know of little exceeding the histologic excellence of the material of Dr. Calvo and others here, but they are still merely describing. They have not manipulated the environments. They are only telling us what they see, and what they see is often what they believe they see. As we sat here and listened to one person "see" a microglia, and another say it looks like an oligodendroglia, I wondered do we have accurate criteria? So I prefer to leave the sarcoma problem, as I just don't understand them.

Dr. Zülch: Thank you. Probably we are correct in saying that if we are to say anything really significant about the sarcomas we need more material. But in one thing I cannot join you and that is your criticism that we are too descriptive. Well, where shall we begin? We certainly can't begin with the discussion of aetiology because there is no way of analysing it at present. Apart from the virus which produces sarcomas, we have no idea how sarcomas arise and therefore we have unfortunately to describe them and go back to the original description of these tumours, because for me at least this distinction between various tumours exists, if you see a brain which is milky and where you see the whole leptomeninx full of cells while the cortex is almost free that is fairly acceptable as an entity namely meningeal sarcomatosis. And this comes true for other entities. Description seems necessary at the moment at least because we want to know more about them. We can't collect characteristics and we would not be able to correlate aetiological agents found in a particular morphological entity, if we have not already delineated it. So I think in spite of your remark we will still meet again and continue describing entities if possible, but we certainly shall keep in mind your criticism that we should not be satisfied with this situation in the future.

These papers are open for discussion. Dr. Sayre would you like to comment?

Dr. Sayre: I find myself again agreeing with Dr. Rubinstein and his descriptions: I was happy to find that he and I agreed on the diagnosis although I was not sure exactly why he said in his little note that this is a microglioma or a reticulum cell sarcoma. I would like to ask him what are the differences between the two?

Dr. Rubinstein: I suspect there is relatively littly real difference, that is why I would like to support Dr. Zülch fully in his agreement with Dr. Netsky.

Dr. Sayre: Some eight years ago I heard a discussion on reticulum cell sarcomas which is unfortunately published in an local medical journal which I doubt whether very many of you can find. The author obtained from the literature a description of a reticulum cell, the reticulum cell sarcoma and a classification of the variations. There was a complete disagreement with the literature on the basic features of this. It is one of the classic pictures of the confusion that occurs in the use of this particular term and I am happy to say that I agree with Dr. Rubinstein also that the microglioma and the reticulum cell sarcoma are the same tumour. We can't divide them as yet. As far as other types of tumours of the sarcoma groups are concerned I have no worthwhile information but I would like to mention the fact that Kernohan is reviewing our cases at the Mayo Clinic and he has found some 16 of these tumours. His classification is not exactly the same as some of the others in that he proposed to call very many of the tumours fibrosarcomas. He believes that some of these tumours derive from the arachnoid cells themselves. He also has a group which he considers to be hemangio-pericytomas corresponding to the hemangio-pericytomas of Stamm. And there was one per cent of both. About 18% of the cases have been from the reticulum cell sarcoma group, 14% of the giant cell sarcoma group. There I think is some chance, when you have 216 cases, to try to subdivide a little as to the different types. The discussion will be published some time next spring. May I say that these particular tumours were stained with every stain at least which was shown this afternoon apart from some of the very specialised stains shown this morning.

Dr. Zülch: Thank you, Dr. Sayre. Who else is going to comment on this? Any question? Dr. Brucher?

Dr. Brucher: I can say that in both of my cases we are dealing with a proliferation of cells of the reticulo-endothelial system. It may be therefore that these cells are impregnated by the microglial method. But the question is, whether this is proliferation of neoplastic or inflammatory nature? That is the essential question, though the clinical facts are very different in the two cases.

Dr. Zülch: Thank you, Dr. Brucher. I think this is really a very difficult problem to solve, and Wilke who has been working with Hallervorden first presented in 1948 a large series of such cases pointing out the doubtful classification of some processes. He thought they could be classified as a line on the left wing of which he could put the blastomas whereas on the right wing ought to be the granulomatous processes. One was always sure to have encephalitis because of the amount of regressive changes. This is quite an interesting fact which one cases see in many cases which have been sent in, the overwhelming amount of regressive changes in the parenchyma as oedema, alteration of nerve cells, myelin sheaths, axons and so on. This is different in tumours which preserve the brain tissue pretty well. But there may be many cases in between, where it is arbitrary to say tumour or encephalitis. These naturally form the essential problem if one wants to see a problem at all in this classification.

Dr. Rubinstein: I wonder whether in the present state of our knowledge when we think of the reticulo-endothelial system we can be so sure we can distinguish between neoplastic and inflammatory proliferation. We meet the same difficulty in the whole group of Hodgkin's granuloma, sarcoma, paragranuloma up to lymphosarcoma in the rest of the body, as well as in the brain.

Dr. Zülch: Thank you, I think, it is quite true. Dr. Sayre?

Dr. Sayre: Just before I came over I came across a report of a symposium on the genesis of carcinoma. Dr. Cowdry of whom some of you may have heard,

was the senior discussor and his personal statement was that it is obvious
that cancers are all due to viruses.

Dr. Zülch: That was the late Oberling's teaching, you know. He has always
stood for that. Well, let's go back then to our point. I think the old problem as
to where the microglia comes from is not solved yet. There is a parallel with
our discussion here in that we just don't know from where the cells come or
what their nature is. Dr. Netsky would you like to comment?

Dr. Netsky: Well, I think we can unify everything. If inflammation is properly defined as a cellular response to injuries then indeed neoplasia is a form
of inflammation. Some type of injury initiates this process and one gets the
cellular response ...

Dr. Luginbühl: I think in the years to come we may be able from the animal side to make some contributions too concerning the problem of reticulo-
endotheliosis whether it is inflammatory or neoplastic. You know that in horses
we have a disease — infectious anemia of proved virus aetiology — and sometimes we find lesions in the brain which I think can hardly be differentiated
from what has been shown here. Secondly in fowls for instance the so-called
Newcastle disease also sometimes produces lesions in the brain which have the
same morphological picture and again they are of proved virus aetiology. Finally we have in dogs the distemper complex of proved virus aetiology and
animals which have been vaccinated may get another type of inflammation of
the brain which can be called chronic granulomatous encephalitis which may
look like neoplasms or like the processes we have seen here. I have quite a
large series of cases already going in that direction.

Dr. Zülch: Thank you, Dr. Luginbühl. All of us are, I suppose, convinced
that very many exciting and inspiring suggestions will come from the neuropathological studies of veterinary medicine. As an example I may already cite
Dr. Frauchiger's book. Scherer also worked on the correlations between veterinary and human pathology. If there are no further suggestions we may
come to an end and I would just make a few final remarks. As I said, Dr. van
Bogaert has suggested publishing them. We plan to publish the papers and
the full discussion with such changes as are necessary and we shall try to
publish them at a pretty moderate price. There is a suggestion of Dr. van Bogaert, that this group should survive as a commission for neurooncology in
the World Federation of Neurology, with the recommendation to invite those
scientists which we estimate necessary for our work. I am prepared to accept
suggestions as to the enlargement of this group, which I may pass on to Dr.
van Bogaert. Then I would suggest and this will be, I think officially accepted
by the World Federation of Neurology, that we have a permanent secretary
and perhaps a collection of cases to which we send, as I said, our problem
cases with our comment. It would be interesting to send those to each other
first and to collect them with the comments. At the end of this session I only
want to express my personal feeling that this Symposium was a very happy
meeting, we have met each other personally we have got interpersonal contacts
and we have learnt our various opinions those where we agree and more important where we did not agree, we saw new problems and we heard of new
methods of work. I think the best feature of this Symposium was the very
frank, open and sincere discussion where each of us estimated each other's
work so highly that we felt that everybody could stand a free discussion without introducing it by a lot of preliminary praise. I close this Symposium then
in expressing my personal thanks and the thanks of our Max-Planck-Institut
für Hirnforschung that you have come to discuss these questions with us and

we only wish you a very happy time in Germany. We hope that you have enjoyed this time here in Cologne as we enjoyed your discussions and contributions. Thank you, Gentlemen.

Dr. Sayre: Dr. Zülch, as the representative of this group it is my deep pleasure to express to you and to the institutions with which you are associated, our deepest appreciation for the opportunity to be present here, for this excellent Symposium, with its varied ideas, and for the pleasant time we have spent in this institute, and we wish to express to you our deepest vote of thanks.

Adresses of the Participants

Dr. *J. M. Brucher:* Institut Neurologique Louvain, Laboratoire de Neuropathologie, Louvain, 57, Voer des Capucins, Belgique.

Dr. *W. Calvo:* Valencia, Avenida José Antonio 71, España.

Prof. Dr. *H. Hamperl:*Pathologisches Institut der Universität Bonn, Venusberg, Deutschland.

Prof. Dr. *G. Kersting:* Institut für Neuropathologie der Universität Bonn, Wilhelmsplatz 7, Deutschland.

Prof. Dr. *G. Koch:* Institut für Humangenetik der Universität Münster, Westf., Waldeyerstraße 27, Deutschland.

Dr. *H. Luginbühl:* Veterinär-Ambulatorische Klinik, Bern, Neubruckstraße 10, Schweiz.

Dr. *W. Müller:* Max-Planck-Institut für Hirnforschung, Abt. für Tumorforschung und experimentelle Pathologie, Köln-Lindenthal, Goldenfeldstraße 21, Deutschland.

Prof. Dr. *M. G. Netsky:* Department of Pathology, University of Virginia, Charlottesville, USA.

Prof. Dr. *N. Ringertz:* Karolinska-Mediko-Kirurgiska Institutet, Sabbatsberg Sjukhus, Stockholm, Sverige.

Dr. *L. J. Rubinstein:* Montefiore Hospital, 210th Street and Bainbridge Avenue, New York 67, N. Y., U. S. A.

Prof. Dr. *G. P. Sayre:* Mayo-Clinic, Rochester, Minnesota, U. S. A.

Dr. *B. Schiefer:* Pathologisches Institut, Veterinärmedizinische Fakultät München, Veterinärstraße 13, Deutschland.

Dr. *A. L. Woolf:* The Midland · Centre for Neurosurgery, Department of Pathology, Smethwick Hospital, Holly Lane, Smethwick, Birmingham, Great Britain.

Prof. Dr. *K. J. Zülch:* Max-Planck-Institut für Hirnforschung, Abteilung für Allgemeine Neurologie, Köln-Merheim, Ostmerheimer Straße 200, Deutschland.